Instructor's Manual for
Brunner and Suddarth's

Textbook of Medical-Surgical Nursing

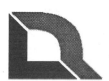

Eighth Edition

Mary Jo Boyer, DNSc, RN

Associate Dean of Nursing and Allied Health
Delaware County Community College
Media, Pennsylvania

Lippincott - Raven Publishers
New York   Philadelphia

Sponsoring Editor: Lisa Stead
Editorial Assistant: Brian MacDonald
Ancillary Coordinator: Doris S. Wray
Compositor: Richard G. Hartley
Printer/Binder: R. R. Donnelley & Sons, Crawfordsville

Fifth Edition

0-397-55265-3

6   5   4   3   2   1

Any procedure or practice described in this book should be applied by the healthcare practitioner under
appropriate supervision in accordance with professional standards of care used with regard to the unique
circumstances that apply in each practice situation. Care has been taken to confirm the accuracy of
information presented and to describe generally accepted practices. However, the authors, editors, and
publisher cannot accept any responsibility for errors or omissions or for any consequences from application of
the information in this book and make no warranty express or implied, with respect to the contents of the
book.

Every effort has been made to ensure drug selections and dosages are in accordance with current
recommendations and practice. Because of ongoing research, changes in government regulations and the
constant flow of information on drug therapy, reactions and interactions, the reader is cautioned to check the
package insert for each drug for indications, dosages, warnings and precautions, particularly if the drug is
new or infrequently used.

Introduction

This Instructor's Manual has been developed to accompany Brunner and Suddarth's Textbook of Medical-Surgical Nursing, Eighth Edition. As in previous editions of the Textbook, the eighth edition emphasizes the use of the nursing process as a framework for nursing practice. This Manual provides many suggestions for learning activities and experiences that assist students in understanding and applying the nursing process in caring for patients.

This Manual is organized to support the content of the Textbook. However, the replication of the Textbook's learning objectives and a content outline have purposely been omitted. The Learning Objectives Section has been designed to provide space for the faculty member to supplement each chapter with personal learning objectives that may be unique to a particular program of study. The section on Collaborative Learning Activities was designed to support the role of faculty as "learning facilitators" who engage students in collaborative learning activities both inside and outside the formal structure of a classroom setting. Team Discussion Questions/Seminar Topics encourage active, participatory student learning, a process that faculty are being challenged to measure under the title "classroom assessment."

An analytical approach to problem solving forms the basis for the section on Critical Thinking Activities. Analysis, assimilation, and data-driven decision making are weaved throughout case studies and nursing care plans. This focus supports the National League of Nursing's mandate to assess and encourage critical thinking skills among students.

This Manual is designed to be used as a workbook for faculty to help supplement instructional delivery. Therefore, an Instructional Improvement Tool is provided for faculty at the end of every unit.

This Manual was written to be "user friendly", to help faculty create analytical and experiential learning activities for students. It was also designed to be a "time-saver" for faculty who are being challenged to do more with less, to do it better and to be more efficient in the process. I have brought a professional and personal perspective to this new format based on 14 years of teaching nursing students. I hope you find it useful and I hope it makes your teaching preparation time a little easier. Please let me know how you like it or how it could be improved.

Mary Jo Boyer, DNSc, RN

Table Of Contents

1

Health Care Delivery and Nursing Practice

I. Learning Objectives:

In addition to the learning objectives on page 3, I want my students to be able to:

1. _____

2. _____

3. _____

II. Top Terms:

1. Advanced Nursing Practice
2. Case Management
3. Clinical Pathways
4. Continuous Quality Improvement
5. Diagnosis Related Groups (DRGs)
6. Health Maintenance Organizations (HMOs)
7. Managed Health Care
8. Preferred Provider Organizations (PPOs)
9. Professional Standards Review Organizations (PSROs)
10. Wellness-Illness Continuum

III. Collaborative Learning Activities:

Team Discussion Questions/Seminar Topics

1. Have students work in groups of 4-5 to a team. Have every team list each category of Maslow's needs and give an example of patient behavior that reflects an unmet need for each category. Have teams share results. (reference page 11 and Figure 1-2)

Need Category	Behavior Indicative of Unmet Need
Physiologic (Sample)	Talks incessantly about food. (Sample)

2. Have students discuss how current changes in health care reform (HCR) are effecting the delivery of nursing care in acute care, long-term care, and community-based health settings.

Activities:

Have students:

- present a topical summary of the latest journal and newspaper articles
- interview a nursing administrator in each of three settings and present a summary of their perspective of the impact of HCR
- create a vision of how HCR will influence nursing practice in the year 2000.

3. Health care reform (HCR) may increase the number of nurse managed centers in the U.S. Have teams of students each develop three arguments to counteract the American Medical Association's position that this movement will not be beneficial for patient care. Have each team use some form of documented data (statistics, research article, government document) to support one of their three arguments.

IV. Critical Thinking Activities:

In-Class Team Exercises

1. JCAHO mandated in 1992 that health care organizations move toward implementation of CQI. Students need to become familiar with the Tools of CQI to function as team members. (reference pages 6-7)

   A Cause and Effect Diagram can illustrate potential causes of an effect so the cause can be examined and corrected. Have students complete the following diagram.

CQI Cause and Effect Diagram: Delayed Medication
Possible Causes

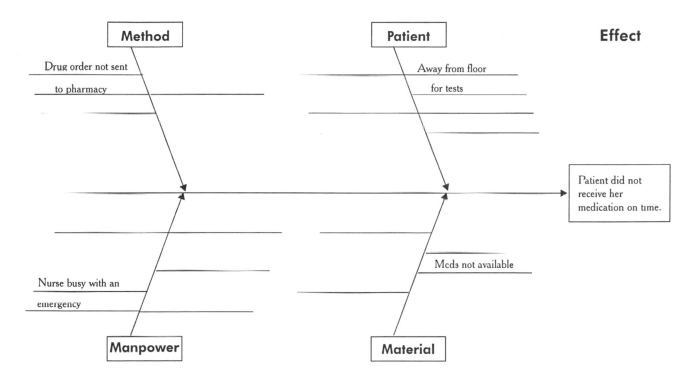

2. Choose one statement in the AHAs Patient's Bill of Rights and have a team of students argue in support and in opposition to the statement. (reference pages 5-6, Chart 1-1)

3

Send-Home Assignments

Gathering data is the easiest way to begin problem solving in a continuous quality improvement cycle. Expose the students to this process by having them construct a Check Sheet. (reference pages 6-7)

What to Observe: The frequency of nursing care events that you observe that can be improved.

Time Period: Eight clinical days

Categories: Fill in your own based on your judgment and experiences.

SAMPLE CHECK SHEET
CQI

Nursing Care Activites	Clinical Check Sheet								
Giving Pt. Information	1	2	3	4	5	6	7	8	Total
Total									

2
Community-Based Nursing Practice

I. Learning Objectives:

In addition to the learning objectives on page 17, I want my students to be able to:

1. _____

2. _____

3. _____

II. Top Terms:

1. Diagnosis Related Groups (DRGs)
2. Discharge Planning
3. Health Maintenance Organizations
4. Hospice Nursing
5. Managed Health Care Systems

6. Nurse Managed Center
7. Nurse Practitioner
8. OSHA
9. Preferred Provider Organizations

III. Collaborative Learning Activities:

Team Discussion Questions/Seminar Topics

1. Distinguish between the role, responsibilities, and scope of practice for home health care nurses and public health care nurses.

2. Explain why accurate documentation is so important for reimbursement for home care services.

3. Describe the educational preparation, job responsibilities, and expanded role of the nurse practitioner.

4. Explain the role of the school nurse.

IV. Critical Thinking Activities:

In-Class Team Exercises

Divide the class into teams of four. Have each team develop a home situation that reflects a safety problem that the home care nurse might encounter during a visit; e.g., a family member is usually intoxicated when the nurse arrives. Have each team present this situation and challenge the other students to develop creative ways to handle safety concerns. (reference pages 20-21 and Chart 2-1)

Send-Home Assignments

Complete the following assessment outline by drafting four specific questions for each heading. (reference pages 20-22)

Assessment Guide

Assessment of the need for continued home care visits for an 80-year-old who lives alone and is recovering from a prostectomy secondary to cancer. This is the second week of home care.

1. The patient's current health status:

    a. _____   c. _____

    b. _____   d. _____

2. The level of self-care abilities:

    a. _____   c. _____

    b. _____   d. _____

3. The level of nursing care needed:

    a. _____   c. _____

    b. _____   d. _____

4. Prognosis:

    a. _____   c. _____

    b. _____   d. _____

5. Patient education needs:

    a. _____   c. _____

    b. _____   d. _____

6. Mental status:

    a. _____   c. _____

    b. _____   d. _____

7. The home environment:

    a. _____   c. _____

    b. _____   d. _____

8. The level of adherence:

    a. _____   c. _____

    b. _____   d. _____

CASE STUDY: AN UNSAFE DISCHARGE

A 72 year old male patient was admitted to your institution with chest pain. He had a long history of untreated hypertension and alcohol abuse. Laboratory studies and serial ECG's revealed that the patient had suffered a myocardial infarction. A cardiac catheterization subsequently showed that he had severe three-vessel coronary artery disease, and he underwent a seven-vessel coronary artery bypass graft surgery seven days ago. Despite some persistent problems with an oozing saphenous vein graft wound and a mild pulmonary infiltrate, the patient is now ready for discharge.

Your problem is that this patient is homeless. It is midwinter, there are three inches of ice and slush on the ground, and the patient thinks that the shelter in which he usually stays is probably full because of the cold weather. The patient seems unconcerned about the weather; with prescriptions and a clinic appointment card in hand, he appears eager to leave. There is a prediction of a snowstorm within the next 48 hours, and the emergency department is full of patients waiting for a bed on your unit. What do you do?

Dilemma:	The obligation to protect the patient from harm conflicts with the obligation to respect the patient's freedom (beneficence versus autonomy). The obligation to protect the patient from harm conflicts with the obligation to care for other patients (beneficence versus justice).
Option #1:	Refuse to discharge the patient, or convince the physician to delay the discharge until the weather is better.
Rationale:	The obligation to protect the patient from harm is more important than respecting the patient's autonomy or attending to the needs of other potential patients.
Implications of choosing this position:	In these days of decreasing hospital reimbursement for underinsured patients, you may not be able to obtain a delay of this patient's discharge if the patient is medically ready for discharge. If you are able to postpone the discharge, however, remember that a delay does not remedy the underlying problem of the patient's homelessness. Additionally, this action serves the needs of this patient but ignores the needs of other patients needing medical care (the patients in the ER who require admission).
Option #2:	Discharge the patient.
Rationale:	Nurses do not have the resources or the power to address complex social problems such as homelessness. The needs of the patients in the ER outweigh the needs of this one patient who is medically ready for discharge.
Implications of choosing this position:	The patient will be at risk for hypothermia, fatigue, injury and pneumonia. That patient's hospital bed will be available for another patient. The nurse feels powerless to intervene with such difficult problems.
Option #3 Potential Compromise:	Discharge the patient with as much preparation as possible to help to ensure his well-being (e.g., a guaranteed spot in a shelter, appointment with a visiting nurse who will see him in a shelter, arrangements for food stamps or meals, a social work contact, a cab ride to the shelter, sufficient clothing, prescriptions filled, etc.).
Rationale:	The respect for the autonomy of the patient, the obligation to protect this patient from harm, and the obligation to care for future patients are the basis for this position.
Implications of choosing this position:	This position tries to meet the needs of this patient as well as other patients in the ER who require hospital admission. The patient is still at-risk for exposure and other medical problems, however, he is less at-risk due to better planning and attention to detail.

Guidelines for the Nurse Preparing a Patient for a Risky Discharge:

1. Assess every patient on admission for the ability to perform the activities of daily living, home situation and social (family, friends) support. Identify patients who are at-risk for an unsafe discharge (e.g., the patient who lives alone and is unable to care for himself; the patient who is confused and lives without supervision; the patient whose home environment is unsafe (abusive family, home is a fire hazard, or the patient has no home)) and make early referrals to the social worker.

2. Advance planning is essential for the patient with a potentially risky discharge. Initiate consultations with the social worker, physician, risk manager, and adult protective services as needed to assess the home situation and begin a discharge plan. A person who is aware of the resources available in the community, for example, a social worker, is invaluable. Be creative in pulling together available resources to meet the needs of the patient.

3. Consult with the physician to plan a discharge date that maximizes the benefits to the patient but also takes into consideration the needs of other patients (for needed hospital care).

Bibliography

Abramson M. The Autonomy-Paternalism Dilemma in Social Work Practice. The Journal of Contemporary Social Work. 1985 September; 66(7):337-393.

Abramson M. Ethical Dilemmas for Social Workers in Discharge Planning. Social Work in Health Care. 1981 Summer; 6(4):33-42.

Abramson M. A Model for Organizing an Ethical Analysis of the Discharge Planning Process. Social Work in Health Care. 1983 Fall; 9(l):45-52.

Anonymous. 1990: Case Presentation 2: The Unsafe Hospital Discharge. HEC (Hospital Ethics Committee) Forum. 1990; 2(4):279-284.

Dubler, NN. Improving the Discharge Planning Process: Distinguishing Between Coercion and Choice. The Gerontologist. 1988 June Supplement; 28(3):76-81.

3
Critical Thinking and the Nursing Process

I. Learning Objectives:

In addition to the learning objectives on page 25, I want my students to be able to:

1. _____

2. _____

3. _____

II. Top Terms:

1. Assessment
2. Collaborative Problems
3. Data Base
4. Evaluation
5. Expected Outcomes

6. Implementation
7. Nursing Diagnosis
8. Nursing Goals
9. Planning
10. Priorities

III. Collaborative Learning Activities:

Team Discussion Questions/Seminar Topics

For each of the following nursing diagnoses, have teams choose immediate, intermediate, and long-term goals for each nursing action. (reference pages 31-33)

1. Activity intolerance related to leg pain associated with prolonged bed rest.

Immediate Goal: _____

Intermediate Goal: _____

Long-Term Goal: _____

2. Ineffective breathing patterns related to altered ventilatory capacity subsequent to recent chest trauma.

Immediate Goal: _____

Intermediate Goal: _____

Long-Term Goal: _____

3. Sleep pattern disturbances related to anxiety associated with a diagnosis of cancer.

Immediate Goal: _____

Intermediate Goal: _____

Long-Term Goal: _____

IV. Critical Thinking Activities:

In-Class Team Exercises

Use Carpenito's schematic that illustrates a decision making tree for distinguishing nursing diagnoses from collaborative problems (page 34, Figure 3-2). Have each group of students fill in the appropriate blanks and compare their answers.

There is a possible problem with Circulation

The nurse <u>can</u> legally order the primary interventions

Nursing Diagnoses:

1. _____

2. _____

3. _____

Nursing Interventions for Prevention, Treatment and Promotion

1. _____

2. _____

3. _____

Medical and Nursing Interventions are needed to achieve Goals such as:

1. _____

2. _____

3. _____

4. _____

5. _____

These are Collaborative Problems that Prescribe, Monitor, Implement and Evaluate)

Send-Home Assignments

Planning nursing care involves setting priorities and distinguishing problems that need urgent attention from those that can be deferred to a later time or referred to a physician. For each of the following patient care problems, have the student circle the **initial priority of nursing care** and write a rationale for that choice.

Discuss collaborative problems that require physician consultation (pages 31-36).

1. Activity intolerance related to inadequate oxygenation.

   Problems: a.   Dyspnea
                   b.   Fatigue
                   c.   Hypotension

   Rationale for choice: _____

   _____

   _____

2. Alterations in bowel elimination: constipation, related to prolonged bed rest.

   Problems: a.   Abdominal pressure and bloating
                   b.   Palpable impaction
                   c.   Straining at stool

   Rationale for choice: _____

   _____

3. Altered oral mucous membrane related to stomatitis.

   Problems: a.   Erythema of oral mucous
                   b.   Intolerance to hot foods
                   c.   Oral Pain

   Rationale for choice: _____

   _____

4
Health Education and Health Promotion

I. Learning Objectives:

In addition to the learning objectives on page 39, I want my students to be able to:

1. _____

2. _____

3. _____

II. Top Terms

1. Adherence
2. Experiential Readiness
3. Health Promotion
4. Learner Readiness
5. Relaxation Training

6. Residual Effects
7. Stress Management
8. Teaching - Learning Process
9. Therapeutic Regimen
10. Residual Effects

III. Collaborative Learning Activities

Team Discussion Questions/Seminar Topics

1. Ask a team of students to elaborate on the statement that health education is "directed toward promotion, maintenance, and restoration of health, and the adaptation to prevention of illness". (reference pages 45-49)

2. Have the students compile a list of health promotion activities that each of them can do, while healthy, to maintain health. (reference pages 45-49)

IV. Critical Thinking Exercises:

In-Class Team Exercises

1. Have students give specific examples, from their personal clinical experiences, of how patient education can:

    1. reduce costs of hospitalization
        a. _____
        b. _____
        c. _____

    2. decrease hospital lengths of stay
        a. _____
        b. _____
        c. _____

    3. avert malpractice suits
        a. _____
        b. _____
        c. _____

2. Have the students identify specific criteria that they can evaluate to determine if nonadherence to a therapeutic regimen among the elderly leads to:

    a. _____ } increased morbidity
       _____

    b. _____ } increased mortality
       _____

    c. _____ } increased cost of treatment
       _____

Send-Home Assignments

Multiple factors influence a patient's adherence to a therapeutic regimen for health promotion and maintenance. Consider a recent clinical experience and identify variables for each category that influenced your patient's adherence. (reference pages 41-43)

Demographic Variables: _____

Illness Variables: _____

Therapeutic Regimen Variables: _____

Psychosocial Variables: _____

For the following nursing diagnoses, develop general immediate, intermediate, and long-term goals. For each goal construct various teaching strategies and expected patient outcomes. Use the following format as a guide. (reference pages 43-45)

Nursing Diagnoses

1. Constipation related to an inadequate intake of fiber and water.

2. Decreased cardiac output related to enlargement of the heart compensatory to congestive failure.

3. Impairment of skin integrity related to full-thickness burns of the right hand.

4. Sleep pattern disturbances related to excess intake of caffeine in the early evening hours.

Nursing Diagnosis:

Immediate Goal(s):

Intermediate Goal(s):

Long-Term Goal(s):

Teaching Strategies   **Expected Outcomes**

CASE STUDY IN PATIENT COMPETENCY

An 82 year old patient is admitted to the hospital from home with a diagnosis of weakness and dehydration after a neighbor found her on the floor unable to get up. The patient has been living alone. On admission she is found to be slightly malnourished, unsteady on her feet and occasionally confused and incontinent. The patient is treated with IV fluids and electrolytes and physical therapy. When she is unable to eat more than 800 calories per day, a feeding tube is inserted.

The patient is pleasant but has some short term memory loss and is occasionally confused about time and place. She sometimes believes she is at home, and she tried to get out of bed once to go the kitchen to get herself some dinner. She is unable to perform the activities of daily living without assistance and has pulled out the feeding tube three times despite wrist restraints. After several consultations with the patient's son, arrangements are made to admit the patient to a local nursing home. Her nutritional status remains a problem since she does not consume enough calories. The feeding tube was discontinued after she pulled it out a third time. The patient's son gives permission to the physician to insert a gastrostomy tube for feeding purposes so that his mother will be able to be admitted to a nursing home.

When the patient is taken to the operating room to have the gastrostomy tube inserted, the surgeon approaches her and asks her if she's ready for her surgery. "I'm having surgery?" she asks. "What for?" The surgeon tells her that he is going to insert a feeding tube. "I don't want any tube in my stomach," the woman insists, "besides, I'm too old for surgery." When the surgeon insists and explains that she needs the feeding tube so that she will get enough food, the patient interrupts him. "I eat as much as I want to. No tube for me, thank you."

Should the feeding tube be inserted into this patient, or not?

Dilemma:	The obligation to respect the individual's autonomy conflicts with the obligation to do what is best for the patient (autonomy versus beneficence). The ability of the patient to be autonomous is at issue here: is she able to understand the pertinent information about the issue and weigh the risks and the benefits of surgery? Competency is the legal term for the patient's ability to make decisions. Patients are legally assumed to be competent until in a court of law they are proved (with evidence such as physician testimony, psychiatric evidence, and observation) to be incompetent and a guardian is appointed.
Option #1:	The surgery should proceed as planned.
Rationale:	The patient is unable to make a rational decision. Her history of confusion and the fact that she has pulled out three feeding tubes despite restraints indicates that she may not be able to make rational decisions. The patient needs the gastrostomy tube in order to be admitted to the nursing home, and nursing home placement is necessary because she cannot safely live alone in her apartment. Beneficence outweighs autonomy here because the patient's autonomy is in question.
Implications of choosing this position:	This evaluation of the patient's ability to make a decision does not meet the accepted criteria for patient competency. A history of confusion and self extubation are not in themselves proof that the patient is unable to make a rational decision. Therefore, if this position is chosen, it may tend to erode patient rights in this institution. The patient may be angry and uncooperative after the gastrostomy tube is inserted. The patient may pull out the gastrostomy tube and harm herself. The patient may experience side effects from the surgery, anesthesia, or tube insertion.
Option #2:	The surgery should be delayed until the patient's ability to make an autonomous decision is evaluated further.
Rationale:	The patient's comments indicate that she is able to comprehend some of the pertinent information about the issue at hand and that she is able — at least to some degree — to weigh

the risks and the benefits of surgery. The patient is showing that she can make a rational decision, albeit one that conflicts with the decisions of her physician and her son. Procedures should not be performed on competent patients without their permission; therefore the surgery should be postponed until the patient's ability to make a decision can be evaluated further (such as consultation with a psychiatrist). Postponing the surgery will pose no risk to the patient.

Implications of choosing this position:

The patient's discharge planning may be made more difficult if a feeding tube is not inserted. Without a feeding tube, she may experience problems with malnutrition. This position tends to reinforce the primacy of autonomy and the protective legal standards for competency.

Guidelines for the nurse caring for a patient whose ability to make rational decisions is in question:

1. Assess the patient carefully. Determine the presence and degree of confusion, if any. Observe the patient's behavior. Is the patient cooperative and able to follow directions? Is the patient able to comprehend and manipulate information in a rational manner? Are there patterns of confusion? For example, is the confusion worse or present only at night?

2. Read the chart carefully and scrutinize the patient's course of treatment and past history. Is the patient's behavior consistent with her history? Is there a reason that the patient is confused or has memory problems, such as drug effect, hypoxia or an electrolyte imbalance? Are advance directives present, and if so, what do they say?

3. Consider if the patient is being assumed to be unable to make rational decisions because she falls into a category of persons who are often subjected to discrimination. For example, is there evidence of ageism, sexism, racism, prejudice against a cultural practice, or a psychiatric problem? In the above case, for example, was the patient discriminated against because she is an elderly female with periods of mild confusion?

4. Consult with the physician to establish a plan of care that enables the patient to be as alert and conversive as possible. Collaborate with the physician to correct fluid and electrolyte imbalances and eliminate medications that may adversely affect the patient's cognitive abilities.

5. From a nursing perspective, ensure that communication with the patient is not a barrier to preserving the patient's rights. Utilize hearing aids, dentures and interpreters if needed to maintain optimum communication with the patient. Consider a speech therapy evaluation, if appropriate. Try to ensure that evaluations of the patient's ability to make decisions are conducted at the best time of day for the patient, that is, a time when the patient is awake, alert and not under the influence of sedatives or other medications that can cause drowsiness.

6. If the patient is clearly unable to comprehend information about a procedure and make a rational decision, make sure that the information is documented, for example, "Several attempts made to explain to patient that she requires surgery for a feeding tube insertion, however, the patient was unable to repeat back to me either that she needed surgery or why. Her comments kept focusing on a friend she had as a child." When it is documented that the patient is clearly unable to make a decision, decision making then falls to the next of kin or the person named on the advance directive. No court proceeding is required.

7. If you find that your patient has been labeled as incompetent but in fact appears to you to be able to make rational decisions, document your observations. For example, "the patient was able to tell me that the doctor wants her to have a feeding tube because he thinks she does not eat enough, but that she thinks she eats enough for an old person and does not think she needs a tube for food." Notify the physician of your observations.

8. When a patient's competency is in question, a psychiatric consultation is invaluable to help evaluate the patient's abilities.

9. If there is disagreement about a patient's ability to make decisions, arrange a patient care conference. If disagreement persists, consult with the ethics committee. Remember, the patient is legally considered competent until a court declares the patient otherwise. If disagreement persists, consult with the legal resources in your hospital about pursuing a court hearing for the patient.

Bibliography

Angell M. Respecting the Autonomy of Competent Patients. 1984 April 26; 310(17):1115-1116.

Applebaum PS and Grisso T. Assessing Patients' Capacities to Consent to Treatment. New England Journal of Medicine.   1988 December 1988; 319(25):1635-1638.

Cross AW and Churchill LR. Ethical and Cultural Dimensions of Informed Consent: A Case Study and Analysis. Annals of Internal Medicine. 1982 January; 96(l):110-113.

Jackson DL and Youngner S. Patient Autonomy and Death with Dignity: Some Clinical Caveats. The New England Journal of Medicine. 1979 August 23; 301(8):404-408.

Jurchak M. Competence and the Nurse-Patient Relationship.   Crit Care Nurs Clin North Am. 1990 September; 2(2):453-459.

Lidz CW et. al. Barriers to Informed Consent. Annals of Internal Medicine. 1983 October; 99(4):539-543.

Perry CB and Applegate WB. Medical Paternalism and Patient Self-Determination. Journal of the American Geriatrics Society. 1985 May; 33(4):353-359.

Wheeler L. Court Weighs Fate of Woman Refusing Lifesaving Surgery. The Washington Post. 1991 February 8: C1.

5

Ethical Issues in Medical-Surgical Nursing

I. Learning Objectives:

In addition to the learning objectives on page 51, I want my students to be able to:

1. _____

2. _____

3. _____

II. Top Terms:

1. Advanced Directive
2. Deontological Theory
3. Durable Power of Attorney
4. Ethics
5. Living Will

6. Morality
7. Nonmaleficience
8. Preventive Ethics
9. Teleological Theory
10. Virtue Ethics

III. Collaborative Learning Activities:

Team Discussion Questions/Seminar Topics

1. Have one student read the ANA's Code for Nurses on page 57. Choose several of the statements and have teams discuss how each statement can be applied to the student nurse role.

2. Review the "Steps of an Ethical Analysis" on page 59 . Ask students to apply these steps to an ethical or moral situation they experienced in the clinical area.

3. Have each team discuss the "Case Analysis" on page 60 and develop a list of additional data that might be included under each major heading: assessment, planning, intervention, and evaluation.

IV. Critical Thinking Activities:

Send/Home Assignments

Have each student draft a sample living will and have the students share the variety of formats as well as the issues they struggled with as they wrote their wills.

Guidelines for the Nurse Facing an Ethical Dilemma

1. Determine that you are facing an ethical dilemma, as opposed to a legal question or a problem with communication. An ethical dilemma is a conflict of moral views, such as the patient preferring a course of action that the physician, nurse, or family thinks is best (autonomy versus beneficence).

2. Gather as much information as you can about the situation and the problem you are facing.

   a. Review the patient's history, diagnoses, course of treatment, prognosis and plan of care.

   b. Assess the patient carefully. What does the patient know? What are the patient's goals?

   c. Determine who constitutes the patient's family (blood relatives and significant others) and their relationship with the patient.
      - Do they visit the patient?
      - Do they appear to have concern for the patient's best interests?
      - Does the family have the same goals as the patient and the physician.

   d. Are there advance directives, and if so, is there a decision-maker named on the form(s)? What do the directives say?

   e. What kind of ethical problem is this?

   f. Have other people faced similar problems and if so, how did they resolve them? Consider a library search to look for articles on how similar ethical problems were handled.

3. Communicate with as many of the principle players in the case as possible.

   a. Discuss the dilemma with the patient's primary physician and consultants.

   b. Facilitate communication between the patient and the physician(s).

   c. Arrange for meetings between the physician and the family if appropriate.

   d. Initiate a patient care conference if necessary to enhance optimum communication and decision-making.

4 If the ethical dilemma persists after the above steps have been taken, consult with your institution's bioethics committee.

   a. Explain to the committee clearly how you see the problem and what you think needs to be done and why.

   b. Be prepared for a discussion of several options for resolving the dilemma.

   c. The committee should help everyone decide upon an acceptable, morally defensible course of action.

5. If your institution does not have an ethics committee, talk with your supervisor about pursuing a resolution of the problem through administrative channels.

    a. Make inquiries about starting an ethics committee.

    b. As a preliminary step, consider forming an ethics study group to discuss various ethics articles in nursing, ethics, and medical journals.

Bibliography

Bosek MSD. What to Expect from a Bioethics Consultation. MEDSURG Nursing. 1993 October; 2(5):408-409.

Edwards BS. When the Physician Won't Give Up. Am J Nurs. 1993 September; 93(9):34-37.

Edwards BS. When the Family Can't Let Go. Am J Nurs. 1994 January; 94(l):52-56.

Fowler M. Reflections on Ethics Consultation in Critical Care Settings. Crit Care Nurs Clin of North Am. 1990 September; 2(3):431-435.

Mitchell C. Ethical Dilemmas. Crit Care Nurs Clin North Am. 1990 September; 2(3):427-430.

Instructional Improvement Tool for Unit

Student feedback/evaluation indicated that I need to improve my classroom presentation by:

Adding Content

1. _____
   _____

2. _____
   _____

3. _____
   _____

Deleting Content

1. _____
   _____

2. _____
   _____

3. _____
   _____

Emphasizing/De-emphasizing the Following Content

1. _____
   _____

2. _____
   _____

3. _____
   _____

Questions students asked that I need to research for the future are:

1. _____
2. _____
3. _____

6
Clinical Interviewing: The Health History

I. Learning Objectives:

In addition to the learning objectives on page 67, I want my students to be able to:

1. _____

2. _____

3. _____

II. Top Terms:

1. Chief Complaint
2. Clinical Interview
3. Data Base
4. Functional Status
5. Genogram

6. Health History
7. Nonverbal Communication
8. Patient Profile
9. Systems Review
10. Therapeutic Interviewing

III. Collaborative Learning Activities

Team Discussion Questions/Seminar Topics

1. Have each team develop a nursing data base that would be appropriate to use in a clinical setting. Include the components listed on pages 70-76 of the text and modify them as you feel necessary.

2. Take the nursing data base developed by each team and have a team member interview a classmate from another team who assumes one of the following roles:

   a. An 18-year old college student whose chief complaints are right lower quadrant pain, nausea, and a temperature of 102° F.

b. A 40-year old mother of five whose chief complaint is tenderness and warmth in her left calf. She has calf pain with dorsiflexion and is unable to bear weight without pain.

c. An 82-year-old diabetic whose chief complaint is inability to walk because of a blackened great toe on his right foot.

3. Use the information obtained from the nursing data base and have each team develop a nursing diagnosis; immediate, intermediate, and long-term goals; and specific nursing interventions to meet identified goals. Use the outline suggested in Chapter 2.

IV. Critical Thinking Activities:

In-Class Team Exercises

1. To obtain an accurate health history, a nurse must focus on four areas. For each area listed below, have each student record what they believe is most important related to the topic. (see chapter as a guide)

Ethical Considerations

a. confidentiality (example)

b. _____

c. _____

d. _____

Communication Skills

a. active listening (example)

b. _____

c. _____

d. _____

Specific Interviewing Techniques

a. _____

b. _____

c. _____

d. _____

Health History Content

a. _____

b. _____

c. _____

d. _____

Send Home Assignments

Complete a genogram or family tree for your family, beginning with both sets of grandparents. For each person, list their age and health status or age and cause of death. Identify any diseases that may be hereditary or communicable. Identify any incidence of cancer, hypertension, heart disease, diabetes, mental illness, etc. (reference pages 72-74, Figure 6-2)

CASE STUDY IN CONFIDENTIALITY

A 35 year old male patient is in your care on a medical floor of a general hospital. His diagnosis is pneumonia. Further tests reveal that the patient is HIV positive and that he has pneumocystis pneumonia, a sign of AIDS. Upon learning of his diagnosis, the patient becomes quite upset but reveals to you and the physician that he is bisexual and has been having unprotected sex with his lover and his wife. The physician urges the patient to notify his sexual partners that he is HIV positive. The patient promises that he will; but after the physician leaves the patient confides to you that he is afraid to inform his wife because of his fear that she will leave him if she learns that he is HIV positive.

Later that shift, a young woman eight months pregnant approaches you. She identifies herself as your patient's wife and demands to know more information about his illness. "I've never seen anyone so sick from pneumonia. What kind of pneumonia does he have? What's his problem anyway? How does a healthy man his age get pneumonia? Why does he have to take so much medicine?"

What information should you reveal?

Dilemma:	The privacy of the patient conflicts with others' need to know about the patient's health status in order to protect their own health and prevent the spread of the HIV virus. (Autonomy versus justice)
Option #1:	Inform the woman that the patient is HIV positive and has AIDS.
Rationale:	The need of the wife to know about the patient's disease to protect herself and her unborn child is more important than the patient's right to privacy. The breach in privacy is considered to be justified by the need to stop the spread of the HIV virus.
Implications of choosing this option:	The violation of his right to privacy and confidentiality without his knowledge or consent will undoubtedly upset the patient and will disrupt the nurse-patient relationship. HIV positive people in general might forgo necessary medical care if they believed that their confidentiality could be violated at any time and without their consent. A policy of reporting HIV status might cause people to lie about their HIV infection. The information you release about the patient may threaten his job, his housing, his marriage and his health insurance. Furthermore, the woman to whom you are speaking may not be the patient's wife; does she have a need to know?
Option #2:	Do not inform the woman that the patient is HIV positive.
Rationale:	The patient's confidentiality is more important than preventing the spread of the HIV virus, and it is even more important than insuring treatment for your patient's wife, unborn child and your patient's lovers. Any breach of confidentiality will disrupt the nurse-patient and physician-patient relationship. The release of devastating information about HIV status can harm the patient you are trying to help. The woman may not be the patient's wife and may not have a need to know.
Implications of choosing this option:	The patient's lover, wife and unborn child will suffer harm and potentially the loss of their lives without the knowledge that they are at risk of being HIV infected. AIDS and HIV infection will spread because the contacts of the patient will not know to curb their own high risk behavior.
Option # 3: Potential Compromise	Refuse to reveal confidential information to this woman at this time but take steps to strongly encourage your patient to identify those he has put at risk for HIV infection. Those people who have had sexual or needle sharing contact with an HIV positive person can then be notified and testing can be encouraged.

Rationale: It is important to maintain patient confidentiality because patients need to feel free to reveal personal information to their caregivers. However, it is also true that sexual and needle-sharing partners of HIV positive patients have a right to know of their own risk for HIV infection so they can seek treatment and change their own high risk behavior to stem the spread of the virus.

Implications of choosing this option: The breach of confidentiality will become a moot point if you obtain the patient's permission to contact those people with whom he has had sexual contact or shared needles. Confidentiality of the patient will be enhanced if the anonymity of the patient is paramount during the notification process. If the patient desires this approach, a health care professional can make the appropriate notifications and refuse to reveal the name of the patient. For example, "a patient of this clinic has tested HIV positive and has named you as a previous sexual partner. You are urged to seek confidential HIV testing at. . . ." The patient may or may not produce reliable information about his sexual and needle-sharing partners. The alternative to seeking the patient's cooperation is to rely on the unreliable guess of the health care professional as to the identity of the patient's sexual and needle-sharing partners.

Guidelines for the nurse receiving requests for information about an HIV infected patient:

1. Never reveal confidential information (diagnosis, HIV status, current treatment) about your patient unless you have the patient's permission AND you have verified the person's identity.

2. If someone presses you for information, apologize for your inability to help, explain that as a nurse you are required to uphold the patient's confidentiality, and refer the person to the patient, if he/she wants more information.

3. Practice universal precautions. Avoid trying to "flag" the patient (ominous warnings on chart, use of more infection control measures than required) which could result in public attention to the possibility that the patient has AIDS.

4. Teach the patient how the HIV virus is spread and encourage him to inform his contacts who may be at risk for HIV infection. Emphasize the importance of early identification and treatment of HIV infection. Counsel the patient about ways to reduce the risk to himself and others. Refer the patient to a local AIDS information center.

5. Discuss with the patient's physician the plan to encourage the patient to notify those at risk from his HIV infection. Encourage the physician to strongly urge the patient to notify those at risk for HIV infection. Remember that notification does not require identification of the patient, just that the person being notified is at risk for HIV infection.

6. If the patient refuses to notify those at risk for HIV infection, encourage the physician to inform the patient that HIV infection and AIDS are conditions which health care professionals are required to report to public health authorities. This may encourage the patient to cooperate with efforts to notify at-risk partners of HIV infection.

Bibliography

Bosek MSD and Mixon DK. Caring for Patients with AIDS: Conflicting Duties in Ethical Decision Making. MEDSURG Nursing 1993 February; 2(1):82-83.

Marcus E. AIDS Patient Sues Hospital Over Privacy; Says Therapist Violated His Privacy. The Washington Post 1991 July 22:D1, D2.

Merritt DJ. The Constitutional Balance Between Health and Liberty. Hastings Center Report 1986 December supplement; 16(6):2-10.

Silverman MF and Silverman DB. AIDS and the Threat to Public Health. Hastings Center Report 1985 August supplement; 15(4):19-22.

7

Physical Assessment and Nutritional Assessment

I. Learning Objectives:

In addition to the learning objectives on page 79, I want my students to be able to:

1. _____

2. _____

3. _____

II. Top Terms:

1. Anthropometric
2. Body Mass Index (BMI)
3. Food Guide Pyramid
4. Ideal Body Weight (IBW)
5. Midarm Circumference (MAC)

6. Midarm Muscle Circumference (MAMC)
7. Negative Nitrogen Balance
8. Polypharmacy
9. Recommended Dietary Allowances (RDAs)
10. Triceps Skinfold Thickness

III. Collaborative Learning Activities:

Team Discussion Questions/Seminar Topics

Work with several classmates and practice physical assessment techniques. Have each classmate describe symptoms associated with a specific illness. Attempt to diagnose pathology based on your assessments. Develop nursing diagnoses that can be used to construct care plans.

IV. Critical Thinking Activities:

In-Class Team Exercises

Have students bring to class a completed Weekly Diary of Daily Food Intake using the Food Guide Pyramid as a reference.

1. Encourage students to discuss their reactions to keeping the diary. What did they learn? How do they feel? Are they interested in modifying their diet?

2. Have students calculate their Frame Size using Chart 7-2 as a reference. Note: You will need several tape measures for this exercise.

3. Have students calculate their Ideal Body Weight (IBW) using Chart 7-1 as a reference.

4. Have each student estimate his/her daily caloric intake based on their IBW. Some will need to reduce calories while others will need to increase calories. Students can use these general steps for estimating daily caloric intake.

    A. Convert IBW in pounds to kilograms (÷ 2.2)

    $$\frac{}{IBW} = \frac{}{pounds} \qquad \text{Example: } 130 \text{ lbs.} = 59 \text{ kg}$$

    B. Basal Energy Needs = 1 Kcal/kg/hr. Therefore, multiply _____ kg x 24 hrs. = _____ calories

    Example: 59 kg x 24 hours = 1,418 daily calories

    C. Increase by 40% for moderate activity levels (for students)

    $$\frac{}{daily\,calories} \times \frac{}{percent} = \frac{}{}$$

    Example: 1,418 calories x 40% (moderate activity) = 1,985 calories

    D. Divide calories by percentage distribution of carbohydrate, fat, and protein.

carbohydrate =	50% of _____	= _____	calories
	(50% of 1985	= 992	calories)
fat =	30% of _____	= _____	calories
	(30% of 1985	= 596	calories)
protein =	20% of _____	= _____	calories
	(20% of 1985	= 397	calories)

    E. Estimate grams for each

    Carbohydrates_____ calories ÷ 4 Gms/Cal = _____

    Fat_____ calories ÷ 9 Gms/Cal = _____

    Protein_____ calories ÷ 4 Gms/Cal = _____

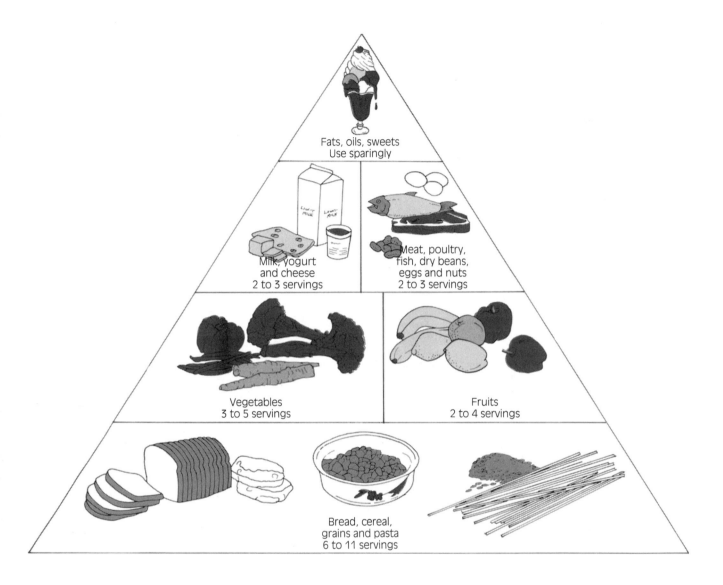

Figure 7-7

Send Home Assignment (con't)

Complete a weekly diary of your daily food intake, listing foods according to servings per food group. Estimate calories for each serving using a reference calorie book. Use the chart provided.

DAY OF WEEK / FOOD GROUP	M		T		W		T		F		S		S	
Group/Servings/Calories	#	C	#	C	#	C	#	C	#	C	#	C	#	C
Bread, cereal, rice, pasta														
Fruit														
Vegetable														
Meat, poultry, fish														
Milk, yogurt, cheese														
Fats, oils, sweets														
Daily Totals														

Instructional Improvement Tool for Unit

Student feedback/evaluation indicated that I need to improve my classroom presentation by:

Adding Content

1. _____

   _____

2. _____

   _____

3. _____

   _____

Deleting Content

1. _____

   _____

2. _____

   _____

3. _____

   _____

Emphasizing/De-emphasizing the Following Content

1. _____

   _____

2. _____

   _____

3. _____

   _____

Questions students asked that I need to research for the future are:

1. _____

   _____

   _____

2. _____

   _____

3. _____

   _____

8
Homeostasis and Pathophysiologic Processes

I. Learning Objectives:

In addition to the learning objectives on page 95, I want my students to be able to:

1. _____

2. _____

3. _____

II. Top Terms:

1. Adaption
2. Chemical Mediators
3. Compensatory
4. Homeostasis
5. Infectious Agent

6. Inflammation
7. Infectious Agent
8. Negative Feedback
9. Psychogenic Factors
10. Ventilation - Perfusion

III. Collaborative Learning Activities:

Team Discussion Questions/Seminar Topics

Read the "Representative Pathophysiologic Process: Hypertensive Heart Disease" presented on pages 97-98. Starting with decreased renal blood flow and ending with fluid invasion of the alveolar spaces, draw an illustration of the pathophysiological response.

Flow Chart: Representative Pathophysiologic Process:
              Hypertensive Heart Disease

Decreased Renal   =   ↑ _____   } =   ↑ _____
Blood Flow   ↑ _____   ↑ _____   } = ↑ Increased
                         ↑ _____   ↑ _____   Extracellular
                                                                            Fluid

Increased   =   ↑ _____   } =   ↑ _____   } = ↑ Increased Stroke
Extracellular Fluid   ↑ _____   ↑ _____   Volume

Increased Stroke   =   ↑ _____   } =   ↑ _____
Volume   ↑ _____   ↑ _____   } = ↑ Increased
                                                   ↑ _____   Pulmonary
                                                                            Activity

Increased   =   ↑ _____
Pulmonary Activity

IV. Critical Thinking Activities:

Send Home Assignments

Have students read the "Representative Pathophysiologic Process: Hypertensive Heart Disease" presented on pages 97-98. Construct an outline of nursing implications and supporting rationales to meet identified patient needs related to three compensatory mechanisms. Use the nursing process as a guide for developing the nursing implications.

(See Answer Key to Chapter 8 in the Student Studyguide as an additional reference to help with this assignment.)

1. Persistent arteriolar constriction results in increased cardiac output to overcome peripheral resistance. Sympathetic nervous system stimulation increases the heart rate, while selective vasoconstriction facilitates the return of more blood to the heart.

Selected Compensatory Mechanisms	Nursing Implications	Rationale
a. Arterial pressure rises in response to increased peripheral resistance.		
b. The heart rate increases to increase cardiac output.		
c. Vasoconstriction occurs in peripheral organs to increase stroke volume.		

2. Compensatory mechanisms reach an end point and then become maladaptive. Adaptive mechanisms to increase cardiac output create an increased work load on the heart. Resistance to blood ejection increases. The left ventricle hypertrophies, dilates, and enlarges. Left ventricular failure eventually occurs with forward and backward effects.

Selected Compensatory Mechanisms	Nursing Implications	Rationale
a. Coronary arteries degenerate, depleting the blood supply to the myocardium.		
b. Cardiomegaly occurs in an attempt to increase stroke volume.		
c. The heart becomes engorged with blood it cannot pump out. This results from the renin-aldosterone mechanism.		
d. Forward failure is associated with low cardiac output plus decreased tissue perfusion.		
e. Backward failure raises end diastolic pressure and is reflected in pulmonary congestion.		

3. As backward heart failure progresses, gas exchange is disrupted. Fluid shifts occur, leading to pulmonary edema. Right failure eventually occurs. The body is in total failure and close to death.

Selected Compensatory Mechanisms	Nursing Implications	Rationale
a. Fluid exudes from the capillaries into the alveolar spaces.		
b. Backward progression leads to congestion in the veins and organs drained by the venae cavae.		

9
Stress and Adaptation

I. Learning Objectives:

In addition to the learning objectives on page 105, I want my students to be able to:

1. _____

2. _____

3. _____

II. Top Terms:

1. Catecholamines
2. General Adaptation Syndrome
3. Guided Imagery
4. Hans Selye
5. Hypothalamic - Pituitary Response

6. Life - Change Units
7. Local Adaptation Syndrome
8. Maladaptive Responses
9. Medullary Response
10. Stressor

III. Collaborative Learning Activities:

Team Discussion Questions/Seminar Topics

1. For each of the situations below, compare your expected coping behavior with that of a classmate.

    a. You arrive home from school to find that your house has been robbed.

    b. The school nurse calls and asks you to meet her at the hospital because your son needs stitches in his face.

    c. Your parents announce their divorce after 30 years of marriage.

2. Discuss the physiological signals that make you aware you are responding to stress.

3. Describe patterns of coping behavior that have worked well for you in the past and that you would use again during a stressful event.

4. Name several daily stressors in your life, and compare your list with that of a classmate. Compare the coping mechanisms each of you uses.

IV. Critical Thinking Activities:

Send-Home Assignments

The sympathetic-adrenal-medullary response and the hypothalamic- pituitary response to stressors are adaptive and protective mechanisms that maintain the homeostasis balance of the body.

Complete the Flow Chart.

Legend: An ⬭ represents the beginning of the process, a ▭ represents steps in the process, and a △ represents the physiologic end responses. Use pages 109-111 and Figure 9-1, p. 110 as a guide.

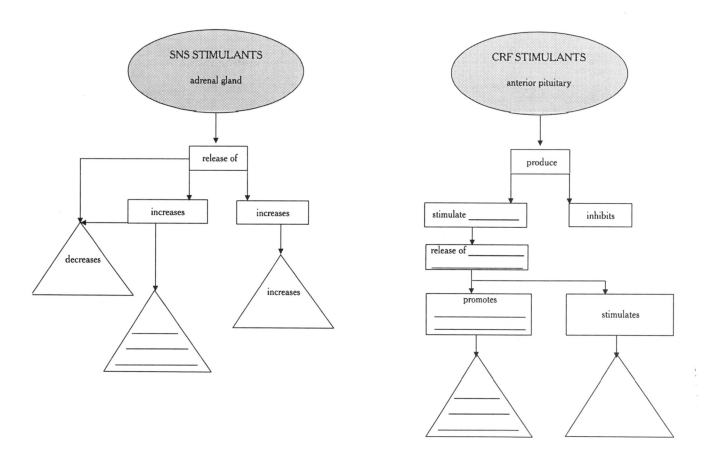

Figure 9-1

36

10
Human Response to Illness

I. Learning Objectives:

In addition to the learning objectives on page 119, I want my students to be able to:

1. _____

2. _____

3. _____

II. Top Terms:

1. Stages of Illness
2. "Accepted" Illness
3. Restitution Period
4. Self-Image
5. Remissions

6. Inclusion
7. Autonomy
8. Control Behavior
9. Denial
10. Cognition

III. Collaborative Learning Activities:

Team Discussion Questions/Seminar Topics

1. Work with your team and develop a definition of burnout. What precipitates it and exaggerates it? What emotional responses are involved, and what coping mechanisms can help? Share definitions among teams.

2. Compare your emotional reactions to an acute illness with those of a classmate who has experienced an acute illness. Discuss the coping mechanisms that helped you adjust to an altered self- image. Based on your prior experience, how would you alter your behavior if you experienced another acute illness? Discuss how these learned behaviors would assist you in coping with a chronic illness. Share the similarities and differences of your team's emotional reactions with other teams.

IV. Critical Thinking Activities:

In-Class Team Exercises

Divide your students into teams of four. Have each team complete the chart below and share their answers. Encourage dialogue about the various stages of adjustment to illness.

Outline nursing activities to meet the expected emotional reactions of a 19-year-old professional ice skater who is diagnosed as having rheumatoid arthritis. She can no longer skate because of inflamed joints. She is at home with her parents. Use the sample outline format provided as a guide.

Pathophysiological Change	Emotional Reaction	Specific Nursing Interventions	Evaulation Criteria

Send-Home Assignments

Interview a family member or friend who is experiencing an acute or chronic illness and complete the following assessment form:

ASSESSMENT FORM

Human Response to Illness

Individual: _____ Stage of Illness: _____

Illness: _____

Emotional Responses Exhibited: _____

_____

_____

Unmet Basic Needs: _____

_____

Self-Image Changes: _____

_____

Current Coping Strategies: _____

_____

_____

List several activities that you can do to promote more effective coping strategies: _____

_____

_____

_____

CASE STUDY: A PATIENT'S DESPERATE REQUEST

You are the home care nurse for a 47-year-old male patient terminally ill with pancreatic cancer. His symptoms have proven difficult to manage: severe pain, nausea, vomiting, diarrhea and skin breakdown. Despite these problems, he has ready outlived his original three-month prognosis and his vital signs remain stable.

On a Monday morning, you receive a report that he contacted the on-call nurse three separate times over the weekend because of his pain, and that his IV Morphine was increased from 40 mg/hr to 50 mg/hr over the course of two days in an attempt to control the pain. When you visit him that afternoon, you find him anxious and in pain. He indicates that he cannot stand the pain anymore . He feels his life is not worth living in this painful condition. He wants to die, and he wants you to help him. What should you do?

Dilemma:	The obligation to respect the patient's autonomy conflicts with the obligation to do the patient no harm (autonomy versus non-maleficence). Another way to frame the debate is that the patient's autonomy conflicts with the standards of the nursing profession (autonomy versus the integrity of the nursing profession).
Option #1:	Agree to assist the patient with his suicide.
Rationale:	The autonomy of the patient in choosing his death and the timing of his death is more important than an obligation not to harm him. Indeed, not to agree to assist him in his suicide would be to harm him by allowing him to continue to suffer.
Implication of choosing this position:	You may face criminal charges and professional difficulties by following this plan. Your advice or actions in assisting with the patient's suicide may injure him but not cause his death. You might assist in the suicide of a patient who may have changed his mind at another time under different circumstances.
Option #2:	Refuse to participate in any way with this patient's plan.
Rationale:	The duty to do no harm and prevent killing is more important than the autonomy of this patient.
Implication of choosing this position:	The patient may continue to live and suffer in pain. The nurse-patient relationship may be disrupted.
Option #3: Potential Compromise:	Talk with the patient and discuss why he wants to commit suicide. Is his pain the problem, or are there other factors — such as a family dispute or a money problem — at issue? Explore with the patient possible alternatives to his pain treatment or family or monetary problem. Obtain medical, psychiatric, pastoral care, social work, or pharmacist consultations as needed to seek resolution to these problems. Explain your reasons — legal, ethical — why you will not assist in his suicide.
Rationale:	This approach respects autonomy by engaging the patient as a partner in solving problems, but also prevents harm to the patient.
Implications of choosing this position:	The patient may continue to suffer if the cause of his suffering is not easily remedied. The nurse-patient relationship is maintained. There are no legal problems involved in this approach, and the nurse does not violate her profession's standards. The patient receives attention to his problems and emotional support.

Guidelines for the nurse whose patient requests her assistance in committing suicide:

1. Never assist in the suicide of a patient. It is illegal.

2. Explore with your patient the reasons he is considering suicide. Frequently, depression or poor pain control is the source of suicidal thoughts for the terminally ill patient.

3. Initiate appropriate consultations, e.g. chaplain, psychiatric nurse, social worker. With these consultants and the physician, formulate a plan to treat the cause of the patient's distress, such as poor pain control.

4. Provide emotional support to the patient and family.

Bibliography

Caplan H. It's Time We Helped Patients Die. RN. 1987 November; 44-51.

Cassel, CK and Meier DE. Morals and Moralism in the Debate over Euthanasia and Assisted Suicide. New England Journal of Medicine. 1990 September; 323(11):750-752.

Cate S. Death by Choice. Am J Nurs. 1991 July; 91(7):33-34.

Singer PA and Seigler M. Euthanasia: A Critique. New England Journal of Medicine 1990 June 28; 322(26):1881-1883.

Yeates C. and Caine ED. Rational Suicide and the Right to Die: Reality and Myth. New England Journal of Medicine. 1991 October 10; 325(15):1100-1102.

11
Transcultural Perspectives in Nursing

I. Learning Objectives:

In addition to the learning objectives on page 113, I want my students to be able to:

1. _____

2. _____

3. _____

II. Top Terms:

1. Acculturation
2. Acupuncture
3. Cultural Taboos
4. Faith Healing
5. Herbalist

6. Minority
7. Spiritualist
8. Subculture
9. Yin/Yang

III. Collaborative Learning Activities:

Team Discussion Questions/Seminar Topics

1. Compare and contrast Dr. Madeleine Leninger's definition of culture (1978) with Sir Edward Taylor's original definition (1871).

2. Explain variations in interpreting the concepts of space, distance, and time relative to communication among several different cultures.

3. Explain the naturalistic view of the cause of illness and disease.

IV. Critical Thinking Activities:

In-Class Team Exercises

Assign the class to groups of four. Have each group choose one of Leninger's terms used to describe her theory of "Cultural Care Diversity and Universality." Each group should define and explain the term relative to several culture groups: African Americans, Hispanics, Native Americans, Asians, and Indo-Chinese. (reference pages 134-138)

Terms to Use:

Cultural Care Accommodation

Cultural Care Repatterning

Culturally Congruent Nursing

Acculturation

Cultural Blindness

Cultural Imposition

Cultural Taboos

Send-Home Assignments

Assign students a project whereby they need to interview a fellow student, friend, neighbor or family member who represents a culture different from their own. The content of the interview can be individually determined. What is most important in the dialogue is identification of communication barriers and methods used to overcome those barriers. (reference pages 134-138, Chart 11-1)

CASE STUDIES IN MULTICULTURALISM

1. A patient with terminal breast cancer is admitted to an oncology unit. She is sedated from high levels of pain medication. The oncologist approaches the patient's husband and states that the patient should be designated as Do Not Resuscitate because of the imminence of her death. The patient's husband refuses to agree to the suggestion of the DNR order, saying that he and his wife are Muslims and their religion mandates health care up to the last minute of life. When the physician hesitates to accept this position and suggests that he will talk to the patient herself about it when she is more alert, the patient's husband objects. According to their religion, he says, the husband makes the decisions for the wife. Who, if anyone, should authorize a DNR order?

2. A patient in her 39th week of a normal pregnancy is just entering the final stage of labor when the nurses on the Labor and Delivery unit change shift. Her new nurse arrives, assesses her, checks for a fetal heart tone and then leaves the room to call her physician, Dr. Edward Richards. As soon as the nurse leaves the room, the patient calls the nurses' station and demands that a different nurse take care of her. She does not want a male nurse. Should the Labor and Delivery charge nurse change the nurse's assignment?

3. A medical floor has only two remaining vacant beds. The charge nurse on the evening shift assigns a female patient admitted from the emergency department to a bed in a double room, leaving a private room bed available for a male or a female admission, or for a patient who requires isolation. When the emergency department patient arrives — a 75 year old white female with congestive heart failure — she takes one look at her assigned roommate and refuses to get off the stretcher. "I can't stay in this room with a Negro," she whispers fiercely to the charge nurse. Should the nurse move the patient?

4. A sign on the door of the ICU clearly announces that only two visitors may see the patients at one time, and only then on the even hours between 10 am and 8 pm for fifteen minutes. However, the family and friends of one patient — described in report as a "gypsy" — have been continually sneaking in and out of the ICU all day to visit the patient, a 20 year old male with a chest contusion sustained in a motor vehicle crash. When the patient's nurse most recently entered the room she found 10 visitors. How should the ICU staff deal with the patient's visitors?

5. An Orthodox Jewish patient who sustained a gunshot wound to the head in a robbery has been declared brain dead by his doctor. The family is told that the patient's life support must be removed. The family, however, refuses to authorize this because their religious beliefs dictate that the patient is not dead until the heart stops beating. Should this patient's life-support be continued or discontinued?

6. The home care nurse speaks only English, her patient speaks only Spanish. Her patient's neighbor, however, speaks both English and Spanish. Should the nurse use the neighbor as a translator for her patient?

Discussion: Each of the above six case studies details an ethical problem that involves a clash of cultures. In case #1, the paternalistic culture of the patient and family conflicts with the individualistic Western culture in the American hospital. In case #2, the nurse is the victim of a cultural belief that accepts male doctors, but not male nurses, in the delivery room. In case #3, the allocation of scarce resources — hospital beds — is affected by the racial prejudice of a patient. In case #4, the ICU nurses and the patient's family evidently have quite different beliefs about what is appropriate family behavior when a loved one is ill. In case #5, religious and philosophical beliefs about death are in conflict. In case #6, the nurse is torn between wanting to communicate clearly with her patient and wanting to maintain his confidentiality.

Guidelines for the nurse dealing with cultural and ethical conflicts:

1. Understand American health care itself as a culture. Identify the characteristics that make it a culture and reflect on how it interacts — for good and for ill — with other cultures. Does it downplay or ridicule ways that are foreign to it? Would you expect the ICU nurses in Case #4 to praise the family that is sneaking in to visit the patient, or criticize

them? Would you expect the physician in Case #5 to state that the family *disagrees* with him or will he say that the family just does not *understand* him?

2. Learn more about other cultures. The bibliography identifies a few sources for information about other cultures and health care, but little will replace the reading of a daily newspaper to stay informed about the events in the world which may affect your patient. For example, a month-long period of fasting called Ramadan may be the reason your Muslim patient is refusing to eat; a war in a distant country may have caused another patient's depression.

3. Make it a point to spend some time with your patient and his family to learn more about their culture. This serves a dual purpose. It will allow you to learn more about their beliefs and it will have the effect of portraying you as a sympathetic ally. Important cultural beliefs should be documented-and passed on, and incorporated into the care plan if appropriate, e.g., "Make sure MD talks with husband about DNR order; patient believes husband should make decision."

4. When making ethical decisions involving cultural issues, try to accommodate the cultural beliefs of the patient and family. Decide, along with your supervisor, which of your institution's practices are really essential for patient care and which can be modified to accommodate the patient's and the family's wishes.

5. Secure the services of an intermediary if needed to help with communication about difficult ethical issues with the family if a disagreement develops among the patient, family and the health care community. An intermediary should be someone from the family's cultural community that the family trusts and who can communicate and understand the health care professionals. This role may be served by a family member with some medical background, a religious leader from the patient's place of worship, or a health care worker from the institution who shares the same cultural background as the family.

6. For ethical issues that remain unresolved, initiate a patient care conference with the family. An intermediary, if one exists, should be present.

7. Consult with the bioethics committee if needed to resolve ethical dilemmas.

Bibliography

Annas GJ. Male Nurses in the Delivery Room. Hastings Center Report 1981 December; 11(6): 20-21.

Caws P. On the Teaching of Ethics in a Pluralistic Society. Hastings Center Report. 1978 October; 8(5): 32-39.

Edwards BS. When the Family Won't Give Up. Am J Nurs. 1994 January; 94(1):52-56.

Engelhardt HT. Can Ethics Take Pluralism Seriously? Hastings Center Report 1989 September- October; 19(5): 33-34.

International Perspectives on Biomedical Ethics. Hastings Center Report. 1988 August-September Special Supplement; 18(4): 1-31.

Marty ME and Vaux KL, editors. Health/Medicine and the Faith Traditions. Book series. Various authors. Published volumes include the Anglican, Catholic, Islamic, Jewish, Lutheran, and Reformed traditions. New York: Crossroad Publishing Co.

12
Health Care of the Older Adult

I. Learning Objectives:

In addition to the learning objectives on page 141, I want my students to be able to:

1. _____

2. _____

3. _____

II. Top Terms:

1. Ageism
2. Alzheimer's
3. Benign Senescent Forgetfulness
4. Delirium
5. Dementia

6. Ego Integrity
7. Gerontology
8. Intrinsic vs. Extrinsic Aging
9. Life Span
10. Multi-Infarct Dementia

III. Collaborative Learning Activities:

Team Discussion Questions/Seminar Topics

1. Work with your team and discuss behaviors you would expect to find among the elderly who are depressed. For each behavior, list several nursing interventions that would assist the patient with coping.

2. List the ways in which various drug classifications can alter a person's nutritional status. For example, antacids are known to produce thiamin deficiency; therefore, vitamin supplements need to be provided for a patient who cannot alter his antacid intake.

IV. Critical Thinking Activities:

In-Class Team Exercises

1. For each drug classification listed, mention several nursing interventions for administering these drugs to elderly people. Cite a rationale for each nursing intervention.

Drug Classification	Nursing Interventions	Rationale
Opiates		
Sedatives and hypnotics		
Salicylates		
Tranquilizers		
Central nervous system stimulants		
Cardiac glycosides		
Diuretics		

2. Consider the following questions about Alzheimer's disease.

   a. The cause is believed to be affected by a decrease in the enzyme _____.

   b. List interventions a nurse can perform to:
      (1) support cognitive functioning:

      (2) promote physical safety:

      (3) improve communication:

   c. Explain the rationale for the following care plan interventions:
      (1) Be predictable in your manner and conversation.

      (2) Avoid use of constraints.

      (3) Treat the patient as a person with feelings.

Send-Home Assignments

Choose an elderly family member or friend and complete the following assessment. Bring the completed paper back to class and share your findings with your classmates. (used with permission, Nursing Department, Delaware County Community College, Media, PA)

Guidelines for the Interview:

(Suggested questions to ask the older adult)

1. Describe a typical day.

2. How would you describe your health?
   What causes you to feel this way?

3. What factors in your life contribute to your health?

4. Tell me about your home and your neighborhood and what they mean to you.

Summarize the living situation:

- How long have you lived here?

- If the older adult is in a new living situation, ask the older adult what circumstances precipitated the change.

- If the older adult has lived in the present environment for a long time, ask how he has managed to be so successful at home. What has helped the older adult to maintain independence at home?

Topic: Adaptation to Aging: Defining Healthy Aging

PLACE OF MEETING: _____

AGE OF OLDER ADULT: _____

1. Discuss impressions, general reactions and feelings regarding your first visit.

2. How did the older adult describe "health" and "old age"?

3. What factors were described by the older adult as essential for a healthy adaptive lifestyle?

4. Identify factors that enable the older adult to maintain independence at home.

2. Complete the "Self-Appraisal of Aging" activity.

Current Age: _____

Projected Life Expectancy: _____

Define health _____

_____

What parts of you are currently healthy? _____

_____

Describe the environment you wish to live in when you are older: _____

_____

Describe the roles you expect to have: _____

_____

What social activities will be important to you? _____

_____

Make a statement of the legacy you wish to leave: _____

_____

_____

CASE STUDY IN THE USE OF RESTRAINTS

An 89 year old woman is admitted to your unit with a diagnosis of pneumonia and dehydration. She lives by herself in an assisted living apartment. She is malnourished, underweight and lethargic and IV fluids and antibiotics are prescribed. By day three of her hospital stay, her serum sodium level is 121 mEq/l and her caloric intake (she needs to be fed) is less than 500 calories per day. The physician orders a feeding tube inserted and tube feedings started. It is now day six. She is on her third feeding tube, having pulled the other two out. The nurse who gave you report tells you that the doctor wants the patient's hands tied "at all times" so this tube will not be pulled out. "Our job is to keep that tube in," she reports. On your rounds, you find a frail elderly woman who appears to be alert and oriented. "Honey, won't you please untie me?" she says. "And take this nasty thing out of my nose! I don't want it!"

Dilemma:	The obligation to respect the patient's autonomy by releasing her from her restraints at her request conflicts with the obligation to protect her from harming herself by removing or dislodging the feeding tube (autonomy versus beneficence).
Option #1:	Keep the patient restrained.
Rationale:	The duty to protect the patient from harm is more important than respecting the patient's autonomy. The patient's autonomy is suspect because she has tried three times to pull out her feeding tube. The physician has ordered that the patient be restrained. The patient must be restrained to prevent the feeding tube from being removed or dislodged.
Implications of choosing this position:	The patient may be upset, humiliated and angered at the continued use of the restraints. The patient may remove or dislodge the feeding tube despite the restraints. Nursing observation of the patient may decrease if the nurse believes the restraints are keeping the patient safe. The physician may become upset that it was not communicated to him that an alert and oriented patient requested that the feeding tube be removed. The patient may experience an injury to herself because of the restraints. The patient may be incontinent because the restraints prevent her from getting up to use the bathroom.
Option #2:	Remove the restraints.
Rationale:	The obligation to respect the patient's autonomy is more important than the obligation to protect the patient from harm. If the patient wants to remove the feeding tube, it is her right to make that choice.
Implications of choosing this position:	The patient may remove or dislodge the feeding tube and cause herself harm, such as aspiration pneumonia. The patient's nutritional status may worsen. The patient may receive trauma to her nasal passages due to repeated insertions of feeding tubes. The physician may be angry that you discontinued the restraints and allowed the patient to pull out her feeding tube.
Option #3 Potential Compromise:	Release the restraints while you are with the patient and take a few minutes to observe her behavior. Evaluate if the patient is able to understand the reason for the feeding tube and the risks and benefits of the tube and the restraints. Explain the reason for the restraints and restrain the patient again before you leave the bedside. Review the chart for the patient's current lab values, plan of care, reason for restraints, and information about the patient's psychological status. Inform the physician of your observations about the patient's mental status and her request for the feeding tube to be removed. With the physician, form a plan of care that addresses the patient's autonomy as well as her caloric and safety needs.
Rationale:	The safety of the patient and the autonomy of the patient are both important, but safety wins out until the ability of the patient to give an informed consent to have the feeding tube removed is clarified.

Implications of choosing this position:	If this patient is alert and oriented, re-restraining her after assessing her may be insulting, humiliating and may anger the patient. Beneficence may not be totally upheld since the patient could still remove or dislodge the feeding tube with the restraints in place.

Guidelines for the nurse caring for a patient for whom restraints are being considered:

1. Assess the patient, paying particular attention to the patient's ability to follow directions and understand the risks and benefits of his treatments. If confusion is present, consider its possible cause. Assess the reason for the behavior the patient is exhibiting: does the patient get out of bed often because he has urinary frequency or diarrhea? Is the patient confused because he is hypoxic? Does the patient with an unsteady gait require a walker or physical therapy?

2. Review the patient's chart, laboratory results and medications as possible sources of information about the problems for which restraints are being considered. Does the patient have a low serum sodium? Is he experiencing the side effects of a sleeping pill? Does he have a hearing or language problem which is being mistaken for confusion? Does he have a urinary tract infection? Is he undergoing withdrawal from alcohol? Consult with your peers, the physicians on the case, a pharmacist and other specialists to help find the cause of — and identify a treatment for — the patient's underlying problem.

3. Consider alternatives to restraints, such as increasing the frequency of your observations of the patient or having the patient's family or friends to stay with her.

4. Weigh the risks and benefits of using restraints. Remember, restraints may aggravate the patient's condition by increasing his agitation, causing injuries, and contributing to incontinence and weakness.

5. Consult with the physician before or immediately after restraints are required. Form a plan of care for removing the restraints. Explain your rationale for the restraints to the patient and family. Document your reason for the need for restraints in the patient record.

6. If restraints are required, use the least restrictive kind necessary, for the least amount of time.

7. Increase your observation of the patient in restraints, paying particular attention to the nutritional, ventilatory, circulation and elimination needs of these immobile patients.

8. Continue your nursing interventions to resolve the cause of the need for restraints.

Bibliography

Evans LK and Strumpf NE-. Myths about Elder Restraint. Image: The Journal of Nursing Scholarship. 1990 Spring; 22(2):124-128.

Evans LK and Strumpf NE. Tying Down the Elderly: A Review of the Literature on Physical Restraints. Journal of the American Geriatric Society. 1989;36( ):65-74.

Hogstel MO. and Gaul L. Safety or Autonomy: An Ethical Issue for Clinical Gerontological Nurses. Journal of Gerontological Nursing. 1991 March; 17(3):6-11.

Mion L. et. al. A Further Exploration of the Use of Physical Restraints in Hospitalized Patients. Journal of the American Geriatric Society. 1989; 37( ):949-956.

Morse JM and McHutchion E. Releasing Restraints: Providing Safe Care for the Elderly. Research in Nursing and Health. 1991; 14:187-196.

Moss RJ and LaPuma J. The Ethics of Mechanical Restraints. Hastings Center Report. 1991 January; 21(l):22-25.

Robbins L. Binding the Elderly: A Prospective Study of the Use of Mechanical Restraints in an Acute Care Hospital. Journal of the American Geriatric Society. 1987; 35( ):290-296.

Weick MD. Physical Restraints: An FDA Update. Am J Nurs. 1992 November; 92(11):74-80.

Instructional Improvement Tool for Unit

Student feedback/evaluation indicated that I need to improve my classroom presentation by:

Adding Content

1. _____

   _____

2. _____

   _____

3. _____

   _____

Deleting Content

1. _____

   _____

2. _____

   _____

3. _____

   _____

Emphasizing/De-emphasizing the Following Content

1. _____

   _____

2. _____

   _____

3. _____

   _____

Questions students asked that I need to research for the future are:

1. _____

   _____

   _____

2. _____

   _____

3. _____

   _____

13
Pain Management

I. Learning Objectives:

In addition to the learning objectives on page 179, I want my students to be able to:

1. _____

2. _____

3. _____

II. Top Terms:

1. Addiction
2. Distraction
3. Endorphins
4. "Gate Control" Theory of Pain
5. Guilded Imagery

6. Nociceptive
7. Pain threshold
8. Placebo
9. Referred Pain
10. Tolerance

III. Collaborative Learning Activities:

In-Class Team Exercises

1. List several noninvasive categories of nursing activity that can be used to assist a patient with his pain experience. For each category, list a rationale and an example of an associated activity. Use the following format as a guide.

Category	Rationale	Example
Relaxation techniques	Relaxation measures help to reduce muscle tension, thus decreasing the intensity of pain or increasing pain tolerance.	Teach the patient to use slow, rhythmic abdominal breathing at six to nine breaths per minute. He can maintain a slow, constant, counting rhythm.

2. Develop a nursing care plan for a 55-year-old woman with intractable pain associated with breast cancer and bone metastasis. She was independent in her activities of daily living before admission for chemotherapy and radiation. Develop your nursing care plan based on the patient's need for pain management.

Nursing Diagnosis: Alteration in comfort related to breast cancer and bone metastasis.

Intermediate Goal: Patient will experience a decrease in the intensity of pain or relief of pain.

Long-Term Goal: Patient will manage episodes of pain and maintain a realistic level of independence in activities of daily living.

Nursing Interventions   **Expected Outcomes**

IV. Critical Thinking Activities:

Send-Home Assignments

Use the Pain Assessment Tool and Visual Analogue Scale (Figure 13-3, p. 185) to assess the pain of someone you know (family member, neighbor, friend) who is experiencing either acute or chronic pain. Bring the completed tool back to school and share your results with your classmates.

A. **NAME** _____ **DATE** _____

LOCATION: Describe or point to area of pain. _____

QUALITY: What words best describe your pain? _____

_____

INTENSITY: Rate your pain on a scale of 0 (no pain) to 10 (worst pain possible)

At present _____ 1 hour after medication _____

Worst it gets _____ Best it gets _____

ONSET: When did pain begin?_____ What time of day does it occur? _____

How often does it occur? _____ How long does it last? _____

EFFECT OF PAIN: What relieves the pain? _____

What makes the pain worse? _____

What other problems/symptoms occur with the pain? _____

How does the pain affect your life and your activities? _____

PLAN: _____

_____

B.

```
|                                                              |
0                          Visual Analogue Scale              10
No Pain                                              Worst possible pain
```

ETHICAL QUESTION: SHOULD DYING PATIENTS RECEIVE MASSIVE DOSES OF MEDICATION FOR THEIR PAIN?

Discussion: Heavy doses of pain medication can have serious side effects, including respiratory depression and death. Patients requiring such high doses of pain medication are often terminally ill patients in the final stages of their illness. Is it right to give as much medication as is needed to relieve the patient's subjective complaints of pain and discomfort even if the high doses of pain medication will shorten the patient's life?

Dilemma: The moral imperative to act as the patient advocate in relieving pain conflicts with the moral imperative not to harm the patient by giving too much pain medication and causing the patient's death (autonomy versus non-maleficence).

Arguments in FAVOR of aggressive medication for pain: The reluctance to give enough pain medication to relieve pain is often based on a health professionals' lack of knowledge of pain medication. Many side effects of high dose pain medication can be managed effectively. It is the highest calling of nursing and medicine to relieve patients' pain and suffering. By relieving pain we act as patient advocates. The purpose of high dose pain medication is to relieve patient's pain, not bring about death. Many patients who receive high doses of pain medication may live longer because they feel better and eat more. Patients with a lot of pain quickly become tolerant to pain medication and may require (and may tolerate) very high doses of analgesics. The obligation to act as patient advocate is stronger than the obligation to preserve life. Most ethicists support aggressive treatment of pain even if such treatment shortens the life of the patient. Patients may resort to extreme measures (for example, suicide) if they are not able to obtain pain relief.

Implications of choosing this position: The patient's pain and discomfort may be relieved but the patient's life may be shortened because of the pain medication. Nurses and doctors may feel guilty that they have caused a patient's death by giving what they consider excessive pain medication.

Arguments AGAINST aggressive medication for pain: High dose pain medication is too much like active euthanasia (the goal of which is to bring about the death of the patient). Health care providers should not be put in the position of administering the dose of medication that causes the patient's death. Preserving life is a stronger obligation than following the wishes of the patient for relief of pain and discomfort.

Implications of choosing this position: The patient's life may be prolonged but the patient may have more pain, discomfort and a poorer quality of life at the end of his life. Nurses and physicians may feel guilty that they have caused the patient to suffer by withholding pain medication.

Potential compromise: The purpose of pain medication should always be to relieve pain rather than to bring about the death of the patient. Nurses and Physicians should aggressively treat pain and judiciously treat side effects of pain medication.

Implications of choosing this position: Health care providers may bring about an earlier death of patients through the aggressive use of pain medication, but patients will receive relief from pain.

Guidelines for the nurse caring for a terminally ill patient in pain:

1. Assess the patient's pain. Obtain a complete description of the pain from the patient including the history of pain, the type of relief desired, and the history of medication use. Refer to the medical record for the patient's history, reason for admission or referral, course of treatment, and the plan of care.

2. Question the medication ordered for pain relief. Is it the best medication for the purpose desired by the patient? Is the dose adequate? What are the usual side effects of the medication and what is the plan for handling the side effects?

3. Discuss the current and alternative treatments with the patient's physician. What are the alternatives for treating the patient's pain? Consult with a pharmacist, clinical nurse specialist, pain specialist, intravenous therapy nurse or anesthesiologist if necessary. Decide on a plan for managing side effects of the chosen pain relief method.

4. Assess if the patient and family are aware of the risks and benefits of high dose pain medication. Inform them about the risks and benefits if needed.

5. Investigate if the patient's status has been designated as Do-Not-Resuscitate, and if not, why not.

6. Arrange for a patient care conference with the physicians, nursing staff, consultants and patient and family if necessary to come to an agreement on a plan for pain relief and symptom control.

Bibliography

American Nurses' Association. Position Statement on Promotion of Comfort and Relief of Pain in Dying Patients. Washington, D. C. American Nurses' Association, 1991.

American Pain Society. Principles of Analgesic Use in the Treatment of Acute Pain and Cancer Pain. 3rd Edition. Skokie, Ill. American Pain Society, 1992.

Bosek MSD. The Ethics of Pain Management. MEDSURG Nursing 1993 June: 2(3): 218-220.

The Hastings Center. Guidelines for the Termination of Life-Sustaining Treatment and the Care of the Dying. Briarcliff Manor, N.Y. The Hastings Center, 1987.

Pellegrino ED. The Clinical Ethics of Pain Management in the Terminally Ill. Hospital Formulary. 1982 November:1493-1496.

Wilson WC et. al. Ordering and Administration of Sedatives and Analgesics During the Withholding and Withdrawal of Life Support from Critically Ill Patients. Journal of the American Medical Association. 1992 February 19; 267(7):949-953.

Agency for Health Care Policy and Research (AHCPR) Guidelines: Acute Pain Management: Operative or Medical Procedures and Trauma. Clinical Practice Guideline, AHCPR Publication No. 920032. Rockville, MD: Agency for Health Care Policy and Research, Public Health Service, U.S. Department of Health and Human Services, February, 1992.

Management of Cancer Pain. Clinical Practice Guideline, AHCPR Publication No. 94-0592. Rockville, MD: Agency for Health Care Policy and Research, Public Health Service, U. S. Department of Health and Human Services, March 1994.

14
Fluids and Electrolytes: Balance and Disturbances

I. Learning Objectives:

In addition to the learning objectives on page 205, I want my students to be able to:

1. _____

2. _____

3. _____

II. Top Terms:

1. Air Embolism
2. Baroreceptors
3. Electrolytes
4. Hypervolemia
5. Hypotonic Solution
6. Insensible Fluid Loss
7. Osmosis
8. Respiratory Acidosis
9. Serum Osmolality
10. Sodium - Potassium Pump

III. Collaborative Learning Activities:

Team Discussion Questions

Analyze each statement and discuss its physiological rationale based on the principles of fluid and electrolyte balance.

1. Confusion can be an early sign of hyponatremia in the elderly. (reference pp. 217-218)

2. Administered potassium is usually retained in the elderly and can rise to dangerous levels because renal function decreases with advancing age. (reference pp. 222-223)

3. Bed rest for the elderly person with osteoporosis can cause impaired calcium metabolism. (reference pp. 223-226)

4. Alcohol and caffeine in high doses are known to inhibit calcium absorption. (reference pp. 223-226)

5. Local symptoms of infiltration of an intravenous solution are edema, coolness at the site of infiltration, and decreased flow rate. (reference pp. 241-244)

IV. Critical Thinking Activities:

In-Class Team Exercises

Read the following case study. Circle the correct answer.

Keith, age 16, has been admitted to the hospital for an arthroscopy of his right knee. He returns from the operating room at 12:00 noon with 750 ml remaining in a 1-liter bottle of Ringer's solution. The solution was ordered to be administered over an 8-hour period. The drop factor is 15 drops per milliliter. (reference p. 241)

1. The nurse knows that the infusion should be absorbed by:

   a. 4:00 PM.

   b. 6:00 PM.

   c. 8:00 PM.

   d. 10:00 PM.

2. The nurse checks the intravenous flow rate to make certain that it is calculated to drip at:

   a. 21 drops per minute.

   b. 25 drops per minute.

   c. 31 drops per minute.

   d. 40 drops per minute.

3. When the nurse inspects the intravenous site, she notes the presence of inflammation. This complication is evidenced by:

   a. heat.

   b. pain.

   c. swelling.

   d. all of the above.

4. Nursing actions for discontinuing an infusion include:

   a. applying gentle counteraction to the skin while removing the needle.

   b. placing a dry, sterile sponge over the infusion site as the needle is removed.

   c. applying firm pressure to the puncture site until bleeding has stopped.

   d. all of the above.

Send-Home Assignments

First, match the statement about body fluid listed in Column III with its body fluid space listed in Column II. Then match the fluid space in Column II with an associated fact in Column I. (reference pp. 206-209)

Column I	**Column II**	**Column III**
___ 1. comprises the cerebrospinal and pericardial fluids.	___ a. intracellular space	I. third space fluid shift
___ 2. is equal to about 8 L in an adult.	___ b. extracellular fluid compartment	II. the smallest compartment of ECF space
___ 3. signs include: hypotension, edema, and tachycardia.	___ c. intravascular space	III. space where plasma is contained
___ 4. found mostly in skeletal muscle mass.	___ d. transcellular space	IV. comprises the intravascular, interstitial and transcellular fluid
___ 5. comprises about 1/3 of body fluid.	___ e. interstitial space	V. comprises about 60% of body fluid
___ 6. comprises 50% of blood volume.	___ f. intravascular fluid volume deficit	VI. comprises fluid surrounding cell

15
Shock and Multisystem Failure

I. Learning Objectives:

In addition to the learning objectives on page 247, I want my students to be able to:

1. _____

2. _____

3. _____

II. Top Terms:

1. Anaphylactic Shock
2. Cardiogenic Shock
3. Distributive Shock
4. Dopamine (Intropin)
5. Hypovolemic Shock

6. Intra-Aortic Balloon Counterpulsation
7. Mean Arterial Pressure
8. Septic Shock
9. Shock Syndrome
10. Vasoactive Drug Therapy

III. Collaborative Learning Activities:

Team Discussion Questions/Seminar Topics

Analyze each statement and present the supporting physiological rationale.

1. In the initial stage of shock, damage has already begun at the cellular and tissue levels when blood pressure has dropped. Explain. (reference pages 248-249)

2. During the compensated stage of shock the blood pressure is normal yet the organs are showing clinical signs of decreased perfusion. Explain. (reference pages 249-250)

3. A crystalloid solution such as Ringer's Lactate is used to treat hypovolemic shock because it contains the lactate ion. Explain. (reference page 253)

IV. Critical Thinking Activities:

In-Class Team Exercises

Chart the physiologic sequence of events in hypovolemic shock. Legend (↓ = decreased) Reference pages 255-257.

Flow Chart: Hypovolemic Shock

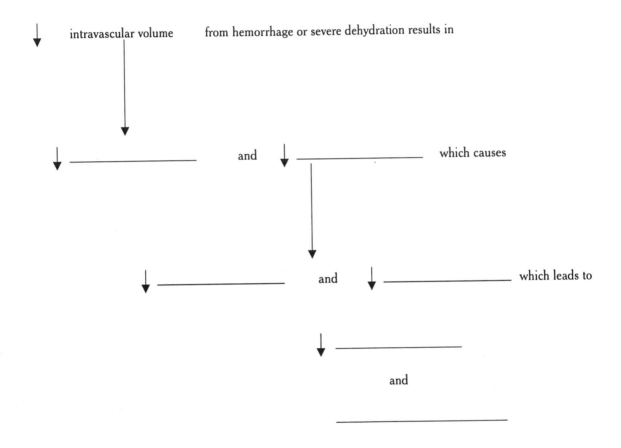

Send-Home Assignments

Read the following case study. Fill in the blanks or circle the correct answer (reference pages 262-263).

Case Study: Septic Shock

Mr. Dressler, a 43-year-old Caucasian was admitted to the medical-surgical unit on his third post-operative day following a vertical bonded gastroplasty for morbid obesity. He had initially transferred to the ICU from the recovery room.

Mr. Dressler had a normal post-operative recovery period until his first afternoon on the unit. The RN went into his room to assess 4:00 PM vital signs and noted that his temperature was 102 °, he was shaking with chills, and his skin was warm and dry, yet his extremities were cool to the touch. Vital signs were 70/50, 124, and 36 and his urinary drainage bag only had 200 ml's from 7:00 AM. The nurse, assessing that Mr. Dressler was probably experiencing septicemia, immediately notified the physician.

Answer the following questions, based on your knowledge of septicemia and septic shock. Reference pages 27-39.

1. Septic shock is most commonly caused by gram-negative organisms. Give an example of a common gram-negative bacteria:

2. The nurse knows that the mortality rate associated with septic shock is between _____% and _____%.

3. The nurse expects that the physician will request body fluid specimens for culture and sensitivity tests. She prepares to collect specimens of:

    a. _____

    b. _____

    c. _____

    d. _____

4. Four modalities of treatment are essential to manage the septic shock:

    a. _____

    b. _____

    c. _____

    d. _____

5. The two most common and serious side-effects of fluid replacement are: _____ and
    _____.

6. A central venous pressure line (CVP) helps monitor fluid replacement. A normal CVP value is:

    _____

16

Oncology: Nursing the Patient with Cancer

I. Learning Objectives:

In addition to the learning objectives on page 265, I want my students to be able to:

1. _____

2. _____

3. _____

II. Top Terms:

1. Biologic Response Modifiers
2. Cytokines
3. Interferon
4. Interleukins
5. Metastases

6. Monoclonal Antibodies
7. Neoplasia
8. Palliation
9. Staging
10. Vesicant Drugs

III. Collaborative Learning Activities:

Team Discussion Questions/Seminar Topics

1. Five-year survival rates for cancer are 38% for African Americans and 54% for Caucasians. Explain why mortality for African Americans is higher than any other race living in the United States. (reference page 266)

2. Discuss the three-step cellular process that is believed to be part of the malignant transformation that occurs with carcinogenesis. (reference page 270)

3. Discuss the use of radiation therapy to interrupt cellular growth. What type of ionizing radiation exists? What cells are most vulnerable? How do radiation implants work? How is toxicity determined and treated? (reference pages 277-280)

IV. Critical Thinking Activities:

In-Class Team Exercises

1. Have students work in two teams and identify the seven cellular characteristics that distinguish cancer cells. (reference pages 268-270) Have each team describe the physiological processes that alter cellular growth.

Cell Characteristics	Altered Affect
1. less fibronetic (Sample)	1. decreased adhesion to adjacent cells
2.	2.
3.	3.
4.	4.
5.	5.
6.	6.
7.	7.

2. Cancer patients who undergo surgery frequently have the four pre-existing conditions. For each condition, have the students list how they would modify nursing care for a patient who has had a radical mastectomy. (reference pages 270-275)

Pre-existing Condition	Altered Nursing Interventions
1. organ impairment	1.
2. coagulation disorder	2.
3. nutritional deficits	3.
4. altered immunity	4.

Toxicity following chemotherapy affects various body systems. For each system below list two symptoms of toxicity and explain the rationale for the nursing interventions. (reference pages 281-285)

Body System	Symptoms	Rational for Nursing Action
1. Gastrointestinal	Nausea (Sample) Vomiting (Sample)	Administer serotonin blockers (Ondansetron) to decrease stimulation of the chemoreceptor trigger zone in the brain's vomiting center.
2. Hematopoietic	_____ _____	_____ _____ _____
3. Renal	_____ _____	_____ _____ _____
4. Cardiopulmonary	_____ _____	_____ _____ _____

Read the following case study. Fill in the blanks or circle the correct answer.

Case Study: Cancer of the Lung

Mr. Donato is a 43-year-old accountant who has been a one pack a day smoker for 23 years. He has had a persistent cough for one year that is hacking and nonproductive and has repeated unresolved upper respiratory tract infections. He went to see his physician because he was fatigued, had been anorexic and lost 12 pounds over the last three months. Diagnostic evaluation led to a diagnosis of a localized tumor with no evidence of metastatic spread. He was scheduled for a lobectomy in three days. (reference pages 290-297)

1. Because infection is the leading cause of mortality in the oncology population, the nurse preoperatively notes the significance of a (an):

   a. basophil count of 1.3%.

   b. eosinaphil count of 4.5%.

   c. lymphocyte count of 23%.

   d. neutrophil count of 20%.

2. The nurse is concerned that the patient's nutritional status is compromised based on his recent weight loss. Impaired nutritional status contributes to:

   a. _____   d. _____

   b. _____   e. _____

   c. _____

3. List five factors the nurse would assess to determine the patient's experience with pain in order to develop a plan of care for pain management.

   a. _____   d. _____

   b. _____   e. _____

   c. _____

4. The nurse knows that a diagnosis of cancer is accompanied by grieving. Usually the first reaction to the grieving process is:

   a. bargaining   c. denial

   b. acceptance   d. depression

5. List four activities the nurse can do to support the patient and family during the grieving process.

   a. _____   c. _____

   b. _____   d. _____

6. The nurse knows that postoperative care needs to be directed toward the prevention of _____, the leading cause of death in cancer patients.

7. Two major gram-negative bacilli that cause infection in an immunosuppressed patient are: _____ and _____.

8. The nurse will also assess for the postoperative complication of septic shock which is not associated with:

   a. dysrhythmias   c. metabotic acodosis

   b. hypertension   d. oliguria

ETHICAL QUESTION: SHOULD CPR BE WITHHELD FROM TERMINALLY ILL PATIENTS?

Discussion:

Some identifiable groups of patients are highly unlikely to survive a resuscitation attempt. Such groups include unmonitored patients with multisystem organ failure, a description which includes terminally ill patients with cancer on an oncology unit, at home or in a hospice. Should these patients who will most likely not survive resuscitation be offered the option to be resuscitated? Or should they rather be designated as Do Not Resuscitate (DNR) without their knowledge or consent? Is informed consent required for withholding treatment? Do patients have a right to request futile treatment? Does a patient need to be informed that a futile treatment (such as CPR) is being withheld? Are nurses and physicians obligated to provide futile treatment at a patient's request?

Dilemma:

The patient's right to choose and refuse medical treatment conflicts with the professional's obligation not to offer or perform futile therapy (autonomy versus integrity of health professions) The patient's right to choose conflicts with the professional's judgment about what is best for the patient (autonomy versus beneficence).

Arguments for designating terminally ill Patients as DNR WITHOUT their consent:

There is consensus that physicians are not required to offer or perform futile therapy. An offer of futile therapy makes it appear to the patient that the futile therapy is a viable option. It is considered a misuse of resources to provide therapy that will not benefit the patient. The patient's autonomy should not override professional judgment about which therapies are scientifically proven to be appropriate or not appropriate for the patient. Patients do not have the right to choose any treatment, just the right to choose among viable treatments. Dying patients expect DNR status along with a non-aggressive, comfort-oriented treatment.

Implications of choosing this position:

Resources will be saved. Patients will not be given therapies that have been shown to be useless. Information about the patient's DNR status may be withheld from patients. Nurses may feel obligated to lie to patients and families about the patient's DNR status if the patient or family is not aware of the DNR order. Patients or families or both may become angry if they discover that the patient has been designated DNR without their knowledge or consent. Some patients may be designated DNR who would survive a resuscitation attempt. An overly broad definition of futile treatment may lead to the withholding of treatment from patients because of a subjective opinion that the patient's quality of life (rather than scientific evaluation of probable success of treatment) is not sufficient to justify benefit of the treatment.

Arguments that patients should NOT be designated DNR without their knowledge or consent:

Scientific studies that describe the futility of CPR for terminally ill patients track the patients' survival to discharge, not their survival of the resuscitation. This indicates that CPR is not always futile for terminally ill patients. The definition of "terminally ill" is not precise enough to justify a policy of withholding resuscitation from patients. Patients' requests for CPR should be honored because their goals for treatment (for example, to live a few days longer to see family member arriving from out of town) are more important than professional obligations not to provide treatment that is highly unlikely to be effective. After many years of publicity in lay press about DNR orders, patients expect to discuss DNR status with physicians before a DNR status is assigned. Professionals should not have to conceal the DNR status from the patient and family. All treatment options should be presented to the patient along with realistic data on chances for success and expected outcome.

Implications of choosing this position:

No patient would be designated DNR without the consent of the patient or family. Some patients would undergo futile procedures at their own request. The public may come to expect that they can demand any treatment, which could become problematic if a demand arises for scarce resources. Some nurses and doctors may be angry at being forced to provide treatment such as CPR. Some patients would remain in full resuscitation status despite the improbability of their surviving CPR. The staff might feel coerced to offer all futile therapies which patients might interpret as viable therapies.

Potential compromise:	Designate patients as DNR when strong scientific studies show that CPR would be futile for those patients' conditions, but discuss the DNR order and the reasons for it with those patients.
Implications of choosing this position:	Patients may still be designated DNR in cases where CPR may not be futile, but problems with communication between professionals and patients would be overcome. Patients may be angry at their DNR status, but they would be given the option of finding another physician to care for them who would keep them in a full resuscitation status.

Guidelines for the nurse caring for a patient whose status has been designated as DNR without the patient's knowledge:

1. Review the chart to verify the patient's diagnosis, course of treatment, current status, care plan and goals of treatment. Look for documentation of the patient's views of treatment. Are there any advance directives (Living Will, Durable Medical Power of Attorney) that indicate the patient's support of a DNR order?

2. Discuss the DNR order with the physician and discuss the physician's rationale for the order. Encourage the physician to discuss the DNR order with the patient.

3. If the patient does not know his DNR status and asks the nurse for information about his resuscitation status, the nurse should explore with the patient what the physician has told him and gently explore the patient's feelings about his disease and his views on death and dying. Encourage the patient to talk to the physician about the resuscitation status. Be honest with the patient. Document the conversation in the patient's chart. Obtain psychiatric nurse, chaplain or social work consultation for the patient as appropriate.

4. If the physician refuses to discuss the DNR order with the patient: inform the physician of the patient's requests for information about his resuscitation status; show the physician documentation of the patient's requests for information about resuscitation status; inform the physician that you will be informing your supervisor about this issue; inform the physician that you will give the patient the information he is requesting if the patient asks you specifically; refuse to lie to the patient; explain to the physician how lack of communication between the physician and the patient places nurses in difficult positions.

5. Talk with your supervisor and consult with the bioethics committee if the situation remains unresolved.

Bibliography

Council on Ethical and Judicial Affairs, American Medical Association. Guidelines for the Appropriate Use of Do-Not-Resuscitate Orders. Journal of the American Medical Association. 1991 April 10; 265(14):1868-1875.

Kellermann Arthur et. al. Predicting the Outcome of Unsuccessful Prehospital Advanced Cardiac Life Support. Journal of the American Medical Association. 1993 September 22/29; 270(12):1433-1436.

Murphy DJ. Do-Not-Resuscitate Orders: Time for Reappraisal in Longterm Care Institutions. Journal of the American Medical Association. 1988 October 14; 260(14): 2098-2101.

Murphy DJ et. al. Outcomes of Cardiopulmonary Resuscitation in the Elderly. Annals of Internal Medicine. 1989 August 1; 111(3): 199205.

Taffet GE. et. al. In-hospital Cardiopulmonary Resuscitation. Journal of the American Medical Association. 1988 October 14; 260(14):2069-2072.

Tomlinson T and Brody H. Ethics and Communication in Do-Not-Resuscitate Orders. New England Journal of Medicine. 1988 January 7; 318(l): 43-46.

Youngner S. Who Defines Futility? Journal of the American Medical Association. 1988 October 14; 260(14): 2094-2095.

17
Chronic Illness

I. Learning Objectives:

In addition to the learning objectives on page 317, I want my students to be able to:

1. _____

2. _____

3. _____

II. Top Terms:

1. Adherence
2. Chronic Illness
3. Collaborative Management
4. Contextual Conditions
5. Continuum

6. Disabling
7. Health Maintenance
8. Prevalence
9. Reciprocal Impact
10. Trajectory Framework

III. Collaborative Learning Activities:

Team Discussion Questions/Seminar Topics

1. Have two teams of students analyze the following statement. Have each team present arguments and examples to support the statement that: "Patients with chronic health care problems may function independently and lead a full life." (reference pages 318-321)

2. Have students identify several recent medical/scientific advances in technology and pharmacology that have resulted in extended life spans. (reference pages 318-321)

IV. Critical Thinking Exercises:

In-Class Team Exercises

1. Have students list the variables that have caused chronic illnesses to become a major health problem in developed countries today. Then have each group of students list how they can intervene, as nursing professionals, to help prevent the rise of chronic illnesses especially among the elderly. (reference pages 318-323 and Tables 17-2 and 17-3)

2. Divide the class into two groups. Have each group debate opposing viewpoints to the following statement. "Advanced technology has greatly increased the survival rates of severely premature infants at the same time that it has made them vulnerable to complications, such as ventilator dependence and blindness." Have students use current articles to support their position. (reference pages 318-321)

3. Have students work in five teams, each team representing one of 5 age groups: (a) those under 18 years, (b) those between 18 and 44, and (c) those between 45 and 60, (d) those between 65 and 74, and (e) those older than 75 years. Have each team present their most common chronic condition and how they manage to adjust to lifestyle and self-image changes. (reference pages 318-321, Table 17-2)

18

Principles and Practices of Rehabilitation

I. Learning Objectives:

In addition to the learning objectives on page 325, I want my students to be able to:

1. _____

2. _____

3. _____

II. Top Terms:

1. Barthel Index
2. Disability
3. Functional Ability
4. Goniometer
5. Isometric Exercises

6. Orthoses
7. Physiatrist
8. PULSES
9. Rehabilitation
10. Shearing Force

III. Collaborative Learning Activities:

Team Discussion Questions/Seminar Topics

1. Discuss a personal rehabilitative experience, mentioning the frustrations associated with a slow but gradual physical improvement. Describe your emotional responses to your illness, from diagnosis through dependency and on toward independence. (reference pages 326-327)

2. Look around your home environment and make a list of those areas you would need to change if you were suddenly confined to a wheelchair. Is there a bathroom accessible without climbing stairs? Can you safely reach the stove or oven to prepare a meal? How would you reach the freezer to get ice cubes for your soda? How would you carry a hot beverage from the stove to a table?

3. Describe a nursing care plan that has well-defined goals and priorities to help the disabled person maximize his abilities and take control of his life. (reference pages 328-341)

IV. Critical Thinking Activities:

Send-Home Assignments

Read the following case studies. Circle the correct answers.

Case Study: Pressure Ulcers

Quincy, age 82, was hospitalized 2 weeks ago for insulin shock. He is obese, has joint stiffness due to osteoarthritis, and has been in bed for the duration of his stay. (reference pages 329-335)

1. During his morning care the nurse notices a reddened area about 5 cm in diameter on Quincy's coccygeal area. To diagnose the presence of a pressure sore, the nurse should:

   a. assess how long hyperemia persists after removal of pressure.

   b. palpate for increased skin temperature.

   c. press on the area to determine blanching.

   d. do all of the above.

2. The nurse knows that to relieve pressure, Quincy will have to be turned every:

   a. 30 minutes.

   b. 1 to 2 hours.

   c. 2 to 4 hours.

   d. 8 to 10 hours.

3. The nursing plan of care for Quincy should include:

   a. keeping the skin clean.

   b. removing pressure from the area.

   c. supplying adequate nutrients.

   d. all of the above.

4. Nursing interventions that would prevent extension of the pressure sore include:

   a. initiating a 2-hour turning schedule.

   b. obtaining an alternating pressure pad mattress.

   c. using pillows to position bony prominences and support the extremities.

   d. all of the above.

Case Study: Assisted Ambulation: Crutches

Rita, a 17-year-old college student, is in a full leg cast because of a compound fracture of the left femur. Rita is to be discharged from the hospital in several days. She lives with her parents in a split-level house. (reference pages 337-340)

1. The exercises that the nurse would recommend to strengthen Rita's upper extremity muscles are:

   a. isometric exercises of the biceps.

   b. push-ups performed in a sitting position.

   c. gluteal setting.

   d. quadriceps setting.

2. Rita is 5 feet 5 inches tall. Her crutches should measure:

   a. 45 inches.

   b. 49 inches.

   c. 54 inches.

   d. 59 inches.

3. Before teaching a crutch gait, the nurse directs Rita to assume the tripod position. In this basic crutch stance the crutches are placed on front and to the side of Rita's toes at an approximate distance of:

   a. 4 to 6 inches.

   b. 6 to 8 inches.

   c. 8 to 10 inches.

   d. 10 to 12 inches.

4. Because Rita is not allowed to bear weight on her casted leg, she should be taught the:

   a. two-point gait.

   b. three-point gait.

   c. four-point gait.

   d. swing-through gait.

Instructional Improvement Tool for Unit

Student feedback/evaluation indicated that I need to improve my classroom presentation by:

Adding Content

1. _____

_____

2. _____

_____

3. _____

_____

Deleting Content

1. _____

_____

2. _____

_____

3. _____

_____

Emphasizing/De-emphasizing the Following Content

1. _____

_____

2. _____

_____

3. _____

_____

Questions students asked that I need to research for the future are:

1. _____

_____

_____

2. _____

_____

3. _____

_____

19

Preoperative Nursing Management

I. Learning Objectives:

In addition to the learning objectives on page 357, I want my students to be able to:

1. _____

2. _____

3. _____

II. Top Terms:

1. Ambulatory Surgi-Center
2. Anesthesia
3. Cognitive Control
4. Depilatory Cream
5. Informed Consent

6. Palliative
7. Perioperative Nursing
8. Pharmacokinetics
9. Physiologic Reserve
10. Reparative Surgery

III. Collaborative Learning Activities:

Team Discussion Questions/Seminar Topics

1. Nutrients are essential for wound healing and recovery in surgery. Have students look at the nutrients listed in Table 19-2 on page 362 and discuss nursing interventions necessary to overcome the results of possible nutrient deficiencies.

IV. Critical Thinking Activities:

In-Class Team Exercises

Have students work together in two teams to complete the following. List specific teaching guidelines that a nurse can use preoperatively to prepare a patient for postoperative rehabilitation. (reference pages 366-372, Chart 19-3)

Preoperative Teaching Guidelines

Deep Breathing, Coughing, and Relaxation Skills	Turning and Active Body Movements	Pain Control and the Use of Medications	Cognitive Control

Send-Home Assignments

In Column I list a common function for each vitamin. In Column II identify symptoms of vitamin deficiency that would influence a patient's preoperative course.

Vitamin Functions and Deficiencies

Vitamin	Column I: Function	Column II: Symptoms Associated with Deficiency
Retinal (A)		
Thiamin (B$_1$)		
Riboflavin (B$_2$)		
Ascorbic acid (C)		
Calciferol (D)		
Menadione (K)		

See textbook chapters on vitamins in Suitor CW and Hunter MR. *Nutrition: Principles and Application in Health Promotion*. Philadelphia: JB Lippincott, for assistance in completing of this chart.

20
Intraoperative Nursing Management

I. Learning Objectives:

In addition to the learning objectives on page 373, I want my students to be able to:

1. _____

2. _____

3. _____

II. Top Terms:

1. Anesthesiologist
2. Anesthetist
3. Circulatory Nurse
4. Conduction Blocks
5. General Anesthesia

6. Malignant Hyperthermia
7. Neuromuscular Blocker
8. Regional Anesthesia
9. Scrub Nurse
10. Trendelenburg

III. Collaborative Learning Activities:

Team Discussion Questions/Seminar Topics

1. Have students divide into 5 teams. Have each team represent a type of anesthesia (general, intravenous, regional, spinal, and local). Each team needs to identify one or more common agents, action and administration, several advantages and disadvantages, implications for use and significant nursing actions. (reference pages 378-386, Tables 20-2 to 20-7)

IV. Critical Thinking Activities:

Send-Home Assignments

List three perioperative nursing actions and rationales for each listed phase of care for a patient undergoing a surgical intervention.

Nursing Actions

Assessment

1. _____
2. _____
3. _____

Planning

1. _____
2. _____
3. _____

Intervention

1. _____
2. _____
3. _____

Evaluation

1. _____
2. _____
3. _____

Read the following case studies. Circle the correct answer.

Case Study: Spinal Anesthesia

Colleen, an 18-year-old college student, is to receive a spinal anesthetic for surgery on her left leg. (reference pages 382-384, Table 20-6)

1. Preoperatively the nurse needs to make sure that Colleen knows that during surgery she will:

   a. be awake.

   b. feel paralysis initially in her toes and then in her perineum, legs, and abdomen.

   c. not feel pain.

   d. experience all of the above.

2.	A major nursing intervention after administration of a spinal anesthetic is to:

  a.	assess vital signs.

  b.	document the time and amount of the first postoperative voiding.

  c.	log-roll the patient from side to side, as needed, for the first 8 hours after surgery.

  d.	record the time when sensation returns to the toes.

3.	Nursing measures to alleviate a post-spinal-anesthesia headache include all of the following *except*:

  a.	ambulating the patient.

  b.	increasing body hydration.

  c.	keeping the patient flat in bed.

  d.	providing a quiet environment.

Case Study: Malignant Hyperthermia

Rachael, a healthy 3-year old is scheduled for hernia repair. During her intubation the anesthesiologist notes that her jaw is rigid and that she is developing tachypnea and tachycardia. (reference pages 388-389)

1.	Based on these assessment data, the circulating nurse prepares to institute emergency nursing measures to treat probable:

  a.	profound cardiovascular collapse.

  b.	malignant hyperthermia.

  c.	respiratory obstruction.

  d.	tetany.

2.	Anticipating the progression of the symptoms, the circulating nurse knows that she will need to plan for:

  a.	measures aimed at reducing body temperature.

  b.	administration of drugs to reverse metabolic alkalosis.

  c.	insertion of a transvenous pacemaker.

  d.	prompt and rapid transfusion of whole blood.

3.	If Rachael had a family history of this pharmacogenic syndrome, it is possible that she would have received prophylactic treatment with:

  a.	antitetanus serum.

  b.	epinephrine.

  c.	aminophylline.

  d.	dantrolene sodium.

ETHICAL QUESTION: SHOULD A PATIENT DESIGNATED AS DNR BE RESUSCITATED IN THE OPERATING ROOM?

Discussion: Patients may be designated as Do Not Resuscitate (DNR) for many reasons, including their refusal of resuscitation, poor quality of life, prediction of poor outcome after resuscitation, and the probability of the patient's demise despite a resuscitation attempt. Some patients who are designated as DNR elect to undergo surgical procedures for a variety of therapeutic and palliative reasons, for example, insertion of a gastrostomy tube or to relieve an intestinal obstruction. Anesthesia or the surgical procedure itself may cause a cardiac or respiratory emergency which would cause the patient's death unless treated aggressively; additionally many routine surgeries require pharmacological paralysis and respiratory intubation, blurring the line as to what constitutes a respiratory arrest. If a patient who has been designated as DNR suffers a respiratory or cardiac arrest during the perioperative period, should that patient be resuscitated?

Dilemma: The obligation to adhere to the patient's wishes about treatment conflict with the professional's obligation to see the patient safely through a procedure to which he has agreed (autonomy versus integrity of the health professions).

Arguments that the patient designated as DNR SHOULD be resuscitated in the OR: There is no firm distinction between iatrogenic and "natural" causes of cardiac and respiratory arrest during anesthesia and surgery. The professional obligation to protect the patient from harm is more important than the patient's right to choose or refuse treatment. When the patient agrees to surgery he agrees to resuscitation. If DNR patients could not be resuscitated in the OR, the OR staff would feel helpless, powerless and responsible for patient deaths from reversible, iatrogenic means.

Implications of choosing this position: This position devalues the patient's right to choose. The patient may suffer a negative outcome if resuscitation occurs, angering the patient and/or his family. Special status is granted to the OR staff in allowing them to override patient wishes, a practice not tolerated in other patient care settings. Anesthesia and surgical personnel are more comfortable with this position (of not allowing patients to be DNR in the OR) because it gives them control of the situation.

Arguments that DNR patients SHOULD NOT be resuscitated in the OR: The patient's right to choose and refuse treatment is more important than the OR personnel's desire to protect the patient from harm. The patient does not lose the right to refuse unwanted treatment just because he agrees to have surgery. The patient's agreement to surgery should include the delineation of all risks and benefits including possible cardiac and respiratory arrest. A patient's death from cardiac and respiratory arrest in the OR is no different from an arrest from so-called "natural" causes.

Implications of choosing this position: Patient autonomy is respected. Some DNR patients will die of reversible, iatrogenic causes in the OR. Operating Room personnel may feel guilty or angry if patients designated as DNR die from effects of surgery or anesthesia.

Possible Compromise: Make decisions on a case-by-case basis, taking into account the severity of the patient's illness, the likelihood of cardiac or respiratory arrest, and the reasons for the DNR order. Obtain an agreement with the patient before surgery about possible limited resuscitation, for example, respiratory and airway support during anesthesia but no resuscitation for cardiac arrest.

Implications of choosing this position: Possible confusion among OR personnel about which resuscitation measures are to be used in the event of an arrest. More time will be needed preoperatively to explain resuscitation issues to the patient and to obtain an informed consent.

Guidelines for the perioperative nurse caring for a DNR patient:

1. Verify DNR order by reviewing the chart for the original order. Ascertain the rationale for the DNR order, if possible. Review the patient's history, course of treatment, and reason for surgery.

2. Discuss the DNR order with the anesthesiologist and surgeon before the patient's surgery and explore with them plans for dealing with cardiac and respiratory problems. Discover if they have discussed these plans with the patient. Ask them to do so, if not already done.

3. If the anesthesiologist and surgeon plan a full resuscitation for the patient and have not discussed this matter with the patient, notify your supervisor.

4. If no policy on this issue exists in your institution, take steps (talk with your supervisor, join the appropriate committee) to establish such a policy.

Bibliography

Cohen CB and Cohen PJ. Do-Not-Resuscitate Orders in the Operating Room. The New England Journal of Medicine. 1991 December 26; 325(26): 1879-1882.

Walker RM. DNR in the OR: Resuscitation as an Operative Risk. Journal of the American Medical Association. 1991 November 6; 266(17): 2407-2412.

Youngner SJ. et. al. DNR in the Operating Room: Not Really a Paradox. Journal of the American Medical Association. 1991 November 6; 266(17): 2433-2434

ETHICAL QUESTION: SHOULD HEALTH CARE WORKERS PERFORMING INVASIVE PROCEDURES BE MANDATED TO UNDERGO ROUTINE SCREENING FOR HIV?

Discussion: The HIV virus is spread through contact with infected blood. HIV-infected health care workers who perform invasive procedures on patients can theoretically infect their patients with the deadly virus that causes AIDS through breaks in the skin or mucous membrane exposure during the procedure. The risk of transmission of the virus from health care worker to patient is thought to be very small, and only six patients are known to have been infected through invasive procedures. All six were patients of one dentist in Florida, who may have failed to sterilize his instruments correctly. Public outrage over the infection of patients by health care workers, however, has led to proposals that health care workers who perform invasive procedures undergo mandatory testing for the presence of the HIV virus.

Dilemma: The professional responsibility to regulate practice based on adopted standards and scientific evidence conflicts with the right of the public to learn if they are at risk for HIV infection (integrity of the health professions versus justice). The privacy of individual health care workers conflicts with the patient's right to know if he is at risk for HIV infection (autonomy versus justice).

Arguments that health care workers SHOULD be tested for the HIV virus: The right of patients to know if their health care worker is HIV positive is more important than the individual's privacy. Patients will have more confidence in the health care system knowing that health care workers are tested for the HIV virus.

Testing of health care workers will also help reduce the spread of the HIV virus by alerting HIV- positive workers to their positive status and allowing them to change their behavior, specifically to refrain from performing or assisting with invasive procedures.

Implications of choosing this position: A small percentage of HIV tests will be falsely negative and will therefore not provide complete protection for patients. False positive tests may ruin the careers of health care workers. There will be the problem of deciding how often to test health care workers, since infection may occur at any time. The more frequently tests are performed, the more expensive the program will be. There will be a high cost of testing for very low probability of gain in safety for patients.

Arguments that health care workers SHOULD NOT be tested for the HIV virus: There is an extremely low probability that an HIV positive health care worker will infect a patient even during invasive procedures. The high cost of testing does not justify the low return in safety to patients. Universal precautions provide sufficient protection to protect patients from HIV transmission. The health care worker's right to privacy is more important than the public's right to know.

Implications of choosing this position: Public fears of HIV infection from health care workers will not be quelled. Money will be saved by not initiating massive HIV testing for health care workers. HIV-infected health care workers will not be identified and will perform potentially risky invasive procedures on patients. Health care workers who are HIV positive and do not know it will not be made aware of their infection and will not know of the need to seek treatment and change behavior to help prevent spread of disease.

Potential compromise: Health care workers who know themselves to be HIV positive should voluntarily refrain from performing invasive procedures. This is the current recommendation of the Centers for Disease Control and Prevention.

Implications of choosing this position: Infected health care workers may not voluntarily refrain from performing invasive procedures. Public fears will not be mollified.

Guidelines for the nurse involved in invasive procedure who is asked by the patient if she is HIV positive:

1. If you are involved in an invasive procedure, stop what you are doing, if possible, or do not start the procedure.

2. Discuss the ways by which the HIV virus is transmitted and the very low risk of transmission of the virus from the health care worker to the patient. Describe universal precautions and explain to the patient how he is protected by them.

3. Always use universal precautions for every patient.

4. Secure the patient's permission for the procedure.

5. If the patient insists on knowing your HIV status and you are HIV negative: you may refuse to answer, citing privacy, or you may tell the truth. If the patient feels uncomfortable with this answer, offer to find another nurse acceptable to the patient to perform the procedure, if possible. Refer him to his physician for more questions. Document his refusal of the procedure.

6. If you are HIV positive, you should not perform invasive procedures that might expose the patient to HIV infection. Find another nurse to perform such procedures. Discuss with your supervisor the best way to handle the requirements of your job, as well as how to handle inquiries from patients. Never lie to patients.

Bibliography

Barringer F. Doctor's AIDS Death Renews Debate on Who Should Know. New York Times. 1990 December 8: 1, 11.

Centers for Disease Control. Recommendations for Preventing Transmission of Human Immunodeficiency Virus and Hepatitis B Virus to Patients During Exposure-Prone Invasive Procedures. Morbidity and Mortality Weekly Report. 1991 July 12; 40(RR-8): 1-9.

Gladwell M. Groups Oppose HIV Tests for Medical Professionals: U.S. Officials' Calculations are Said to Overstate Patients' Risk of Infection. The Washington Post. 1991 February 22:A6.

Gostin L. HIV-infected Physicians and the Practice of Seriously Invasive Procedures. Hastings Center Report. 1989 January-February; 19(1): 32-39.

"I Blame... Every Single One of You": Dying Florida Woman with AIDS Faults Dentist, Agency in Letter. The Washington Post. 1991 July 22:A3.

Kantrowitz B. et. al. Doctors and AIDS: Should patients and doctors have the right to know each other's HIV status? A pair of new cases in Minneapolis reignites the debate while the first victim of doctor-to-patient transmission lies dying. Newsweek. 1991 July 1:49-57.

Pianin E. Amendment Requires AIDS Disclosure: Senate Sets Penalties for Medical Workers. The Washington Post. 1991 July 19:A1.

Sacks JJ. AIDS in a Surgeon. New England Journal of Medicine. 1985 October 17; 323(16):1017-1018.

21

Postoperative Nursing Management

I. Learning Objectives:

In addition to the learning objectives on page 391, I want my students to be able to:

1. _____

2. _____

3. _____

II. Top Terms:

1. Atelectasis
2. Dehiscence
3. Embolus
4. Evisceration
5. Hypoxemia
6. Intrathecal Infusion
7. Keloid

8. Paralytic Ileus
9. Patency
10. Phlebothrombosis
11. Post-Anesthesia Care Unit (PACU)
12. Proliferative Phase
13. Serosanguineous
14. Toxic Delirium

III. Collaborative Learning Activities:

Team Discussion Questions/Seminar Topics

1. Have students outline collaborative nursing interventions for maintaining adequate tissue perfusion. List supporting rationales for nursing actions. (reference page 402)

2. Have students discuss the gerontologic considerations related to the postoperative management of a patient with deep vein thrombosis. (reference pages 405-407, Figure 21-4)

IV. Critical Thinking Activities:

In-Class Team Exercises

1. For each of the nursing diagnoses listed below, state one patient goal, measurement criteria and two nursing interventions for assisting the patient toward goal achievement.

    a. Nursing Diagnosis:Ineffective airway clearance related to the depressant effects of medications and anesthetic agents

    Goal and Criteria:

    _____

    _____

    _____

    Nursing Interventions:

    _____

    _____

    _____

    b. Nursing Diagnosis: Pain and other postoperative discomforts

    Goal and Criteria:

    _____

    _____

    _____

    Nursing Interventions:

    _____

    _____

    _____

    c. Nursing Diagnosis: Alteration in tissue perfusion, systemic, secondary to hypovolemia, peripheral blood pooling, and possible vasoconstriction.

    Goal and Criteria:

    _____

    _____

    _____

    Nursing Interventions

    _____

    _____

    _____

    d. Nursing Diagnosis: Potential fluid volume deficit

    Goal and Criteria:

    _____

    _____

Nursing Interventions:

_____

_____

_____

Send-Home Assignments

Most surgical patients have a nursing diagnosis of impaired skin integrity related to the surgical incision. Patient goals for this nursing diagnosis are evidenced by participation in self-care and the ability to identify initial symptoms of hematoma and infection. Describe four areas of patient education for care of a wound before suture removal.

a. _____

b. _____

c. _____

d. _____

Case Study: Hypovolemic Shock

Fred is admitted to the emergency department with a diagnosis of hypovolemic shock secondary to a 30 percent blood volume loss resulting from a motorcycle accident. (reference pages 403-405)

1. A primary nursing objective is to:

   a. administer vasopressors.

   b. ensure a patent airway.

   c. minimize energy expenditure.

   d. provide external warmth.

2. With a diagnosis of hypovolemic shock, the nurse expects to assess all of the following *except*:

   a. a decreased and concentrated urinary output.

   b. an elevated central venous pressure reading.

   c. hypotension with a small pulse pressure.

   d. tachycardia and a thready pulse.

3. The nurse takes blood pressure readings every 5 minutes. She knows that shock is well advanced when the systolic reading drops below:

   a. 90 mm Hg.

   b. 100 mm Hg.

   c. 110 mm Hg.

   d. 120 mm Hg.

4. A urinary catheter is inserted to measure hourly output. The nurse knows that inadequate volume replacement is reflected by an output less than:

    a.   30 ml/hr.

    b.   50 ml/hr.

    c.   80 ml/hr.

    d.   100 ml/hr.

5. The physician prescribes a crystalloid solution to be administered to restore blood volume. The nurse knows that a crystalloid solution is:

    a.   a blood transfusion.

    b.   lactated Ringer's solution.

    c.   plasma or a plasma substitute.

    d.   serum albumin.

Instructional Improvement Tool for Unit

Student feedback/evaluation indicated that I need to improve my classroom presentation by:

Adding Content

1. _____

   _____

2. _____

   _____

3. _____

   _____

Deleting Content

1. _____

   _____

2. _____

   _____

3. _____

   _____

Emphasizing/De-emphasizing the Following Content

1. _____

   _____

2. _____

   _____

3. _____

   _____

Questions students asked that I need to research for the future are:

1. _____

   _____

   _____

2. _____

   _____

3. _____

   _____

22
Assessment of Respiratory Function

I. Learning Objectives:

In addition to the learning objectives on page 429, I want my students to be able to:

1. _____

2. _____

3. _____

II. Top Terms:

1. Alveoli
2. Conchae
3. Crackles
4. Cyanosis
5. Dyspnea
6. Gallium Scan
7. Hematemesis
8. Hering-Breuer Reflex
9. Hypoxia
10. Olfactory
11. Orthopnea
12. Partial Pressure
13. Rales
14. Rhinitis
15. Rhonchi
16. Surfactant
17. Tachypnea
18. Tactile Fremitus
19. Wheezes

III. Collaborative Learning Activities:

Team Discussion Questions/Seminar Topics

1. Compare and contrast the various respiratory processes: ventilation, perfusion, diffusion, and shunting. Explain the relationship of the pulmonary circulation to these processes.

2. Explain the differences and clinical significance between the various adventitious breath sounds: crackles, rales, rhonchi, wheezes, and pleural friction rub.

IV. Critical Thinking Activities:

In-Class Team Exercises

Assign students to teams of four. Have each student assess the breath sounds of three of his/her classmates. Complete the following chart, identifying as many characteristics as possible. (reference pages 446-448 and Table 22-3)

	Description of Sound, in your words.	Sound Duration	Locations of Various Intensities	Expiratory Sound Intensity	Expiratory Sound Pitch
Vesicular					
Broncho-Vesicular					
Bronchial					
Tracheal					

Send-Home Assignments

Review Figure 22-10 below and explain, in your own words, what the oxygen-hemoglobin dissociation curve depicts and then explain expected changes with clinical conditions. (reference pages 439-440 and Figure 22-10)

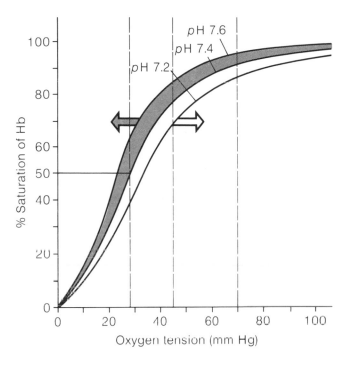

Figure 22-10 Oxygen-hemoglobin dissociation curve. The oxygen can attach to the hemoglobin more easily (higher SaO_2 per PO_2) but has trouble coming off the hemoglobin at the tissues (less tissue oxygenation). Decreased oxygen affinity (shift to right) means that it is more difficult for the oxygen to attach to the hemoglobin (lower SaO_2 per PO_2), but it cancome off at the tissues more easily. P_{50} is normally 27mmHg. A shift to the right gives a higher P_{50}; a shift to the left gives a lower P_{50}.

Explain the oxygen-hemoglobin dissociation curve in your own words: _____

_____

_____

_____

For each of the following conditions, describe expected shifts in the curve and give the pathophysiological reasons why they occur.

Condition Causing Tissue Hypoxia	Expected Shift in the Curve	Physiological Rationale
Cardiac Dysrhythmias		
Bronchospasm		
Aspiration		
Hypotension		

23

Management of Patients with Conditions of the Upper Respiratory Tract

I. Learning Objectives:

In addition to the learning objectives on page 461, I want my students to be able to:

1. _____

2. _____

3. _____

II. Top Terms:

1. Dysphasia
2. Epistaxis
3. Heimlich Maneuver
4. Herpes Simplex
5. Laryngectomy
6. Nasal Polyps
7. Pharyngitis
8. Rhinitis

III. Collaborative Learning Activities:

Team Discussion Questions/Seminar Topics

1. Describe what an individual should do to help someone who has a nosebleed. What indicators would be used to determine when a person should go to the emergency room?

2. Describe the appearance of a herpes simplex canker sore. Why does it appear? What are common preventive measures and treatment modalities? How can its spread be contained?

3. Encourage several members of the class to describe their personal experiences with acute or chronic sinusitis. What were their symptoms? How do they manage to control and treat the disorder and carry on with their home and school responsibilities? Ask if anyone who has had surgery for this condition would share his/her experiences.

IV. Critical Thinking Activities:

In-Class Team Exercises

1.   Assign students to a partner and have each student demonstrate the Heimlich maneuver on his/her partner. (reference pages 472-473 and Figure 23-5)

2.   Assign the students to two teams. Have each team design a poster for the College/School bulletin board. The first poster should include information for students about recognizing and preventing upper respiratory tract infections. The second poster should include information about the symptoms of the "common cold", recognizable symptoms, and measures to prevent its spread. (reference page 462)

Send-Home Assignments

Read the following case study. Fill in the blanks or circle the correct answer.

Case Study: The Common Cold

Carol, a 28-year-old bank teller, felt very lethargic when she went to work on Monday. Her symptoms of fatigue were vague but her muscles ached and she had a headache. By the afternoon, she had nasal congestion, a sore throat, and chills. Two of her co-workers, feeling the same way, had gone home earlier. Carol decided to stay at work because she felt she "just had a cold." (reference page 462)

1. Based on your knowledge about the common cold, list eight characteristic symptoms that Carol might experience.

    a. _____   e. _____

    b. _____   f. _____

    c. _____   g. _____

    d. _____   h. _____

2. Carol's virus is highly contagious because the virus is shed for _____ (hours/days) before symptoms appear.

    a. 48 hours.

    b. 72 hours.

    c. 5 days.

    d. 7 days.

3. Carol's decision to stay at work could cause the virus' spread to her co-workers. Statistics tell us that colds account for _____ percent of all work absences.

    a. 10

    b. 25

    c. 30

    d. 50

4. In the United States, waves of colds tend to appear seasonally, especially in:

    a. January.

    b. April.

    c. September.

    d. all of the above.

5. Carol should know that her symptoms will last about:

    a. 2 to 4 days.

    b. 3 to 9 days.

    c. 4 to 10 days.

    d. 5 to 14 days.

6. Carol knows that the best treatment measures include five "at-home" therapies:

    a. _____   d. _____

    b. _____   e. _____

    c. _____

7. Carol calls her physician and requests an antibiotic. The physician: _____

_____

24

Management of Patients with Conditions of the Chest and Lower Respiratory Tract

I. Learning Objectives:

In addition to the learning objectives on page 479, I want my students to be able to:

1. _____

2. _____

3. _____

II. Top Terms:

1. Atelectasis
2. Barrel Chest
3. Empyema
4. Ghon Tubercule
5. Lung Abscess
6. Panlobular
7. Parenchyma
8. Parietal Pleural
9. Pericardial Effusion
10. Pleural Effusion
11. Pneumoconiosis
12. Pneumonia
13. Pneumothorax
14. Superinfection

III. Collaborative Learning Activities:
Team Discussion Questions/Seminar Topics

1. Explain the pathophysiology of bacterial pneumonia from the initial inflammatory reaction to arterial hypoxemia.

2. Describe the clinical symptoms of a hospitalized patient who would be developing bacterial pneumonia.

3. Explain the pathophysiology, clinical manifestations, diagnostic evaluation, medical management and nursing interventions for a patient with cardiac tamponade.

IV. Critical Thinking Activities:

In-Class Team Exercises

Complete the following chart comparing the various types of commonly encountered pneumonias. (reference pages 481-485 and Table 24-1)

Bacterial Pneumonias	Responsible Organism	Incidence	Clinical Features	Treatment	Nursing Considerations
Streptococcal Pneumonia					
Staphylococcal Pneumonia					
Klebsiella Pneumonia					
Pseudomonas Pneumonia					

Bacterial Pneumonias	Responsible Organism	Incidence	Clinical Features	Treatment	Nursing Considerations
Haemophilus Pneumonia					
Mycoplasma Pneumonia					
Viral Pneumonia					
Fungal Pneumonia					
Legionnaire's Disease					

Send-Home Assignments

Read the following case study. Fill in the blanks or circle the correct answer.

Case Study : Tuberculosis

Mr. McCall, a 67-year-old retired baker and pastry chef, is admitted to the clinical area for confirmation of suspected tuberculosis. He is anorexic and fatigued and suffers with "indigestion." His temperature is slightly elevated every afternoon. (reference pages 495-501)

1. Mr. McCall's Mantoux tuberculin test yields an induration of 10 mm. This result is interpreted as indicating that:

   a. active disease is present.

   b. he has had contact with the tubercle bacillus.

   c. preventive treatment should be initiated.

   d. the reaction is doubtful and should be repeated.

2. After Mr. McCall has undergone a series of additional tests, the diagnosis is confirmed by:

   a. a chest x-ray.

   b. acid-fast bacilli in a sputum smear.

   c. a positive multiple-puncture skin test.

   d. repeated Mantoux tests that yield indurations of 10 mm or greater.

3. Mr. McCall is started on a multiple-drug regimen. Nursing management includes observing for ototoxicity and nephrotoxicity when _____ is used.

   a. ethambutol

   b. isoniazid

   c. rifampin

   d. streptomycin

4. Mr. McCall needs to know that the average length of time for effective chemotherapy is:

   a. 3 to 6 months.

   b. 9 to 12 months.

   c. 2 to 3 years.

   d. 4 to 6 years.

5. The nurse is aware that after chemotherapy is initiated, respiratory isolation is usually discontinued in:

    a. 48 to 72 hours.

    b. about 1 week.

    c. 2 weeks.

    d. about 1 month.

6. Mr. McCall is informed that he will no longer be considered infectious when:

    a. repeat Mantoux tests are negative.

    b. serial chest x-rays show improvement.

    c. two consecutive sputum specimens are negative.

    d. all of the above parameters are met.

25
Respiratory Care Modalities

I. Learning Objectives:

In addition to the learning objectives on page 543, I want my students to be able to:

1. _____

2. _____

3. _____

II. Top Terms:

1. COPD
2. Diaphragmatic Breathing
3. Hypoxemia
4. Hypoxia
5. Incentive Spirometry
6. Intubation
7. IPPB

8. Lobectomy
9. Oxygen Toxicity
10. PEEP
11. Pulse Oximetry
12. Tracheostomy
13. Ventilator
14. Wedge Resection

III. Collaborative Learning Activities:

Team Discussion Questions/Seminar Topics

1. Compare and contrast the purpose, use and nursing management of Intermittent Positive-Pressure Breathing versus Incentive Spirometry.

2. Explain the rationale for administering low concentrations of oxygen to patients with chronic obstructive pulmonary disease.

3. Develop a patient teaching guide for a patient who needs to understand diaphragmatic breathing. Have a member of the class demonstrate how to do the breathing.

IV. Critical Thinking Activities:

In-Class Team Exercises

1. Complete the following chart comparing the various types of oxygen administration devices. (reference pages 545-547 and Table 25-1)

Oxygen Device	Flow Rate	Advantages	Disadvantages	Nursing Teaching Points
Cannula				
Catheter				
Simple Mask				
Partial Rebreather Mask				
Non-Rebreather Mask				
Venturi				
Face Tent				
T-Piece Briggs				

2. Assign students to groups of 6. Have one student in each group demonstrate four postural drainage positions while other team members explain the lobes being drained by each position (reference pages 547-549 and Figure 25-3)

3. Assign students to groups of 4. Identify a team leader who will demonstrate the proper technique of percussion and vibration. (reference pages 549-550 and Figure 25-4)

107

Send-Home Assignments

Develop a nursing care plan for each of the following situations, which involve managing a patient on mechanical ventilation.

Richard, age 19, has been managed on a volume-controlled ventilator for several weeks after being admitted for drug overdose associated with alcohol intake. Before admission, Richard was a school athlete who was in good health and not known to use drugs or drink alcoholic beverages to extreme. (reference pages 555-564)

Nursing Diagnosis: Ineffective breathing patterns related to physiological insult to respiratory function

Immediate Goal(s):

Intermediate Goal(s):

Long-Term Goal(s):

Nursing Interventions   **Expected Outcomes**

2. Sally, a 69-year-old patient with emphysema, has been managed on a ventilator since her pneumonectomy 3 weeks ago. Sally had surgery for carcinoma of the right lung. Her emphysema was believed to be related to a history of smoking two packs of cigarettes a day for the past 40 years. (reference pages 555-564)

Nursing Diagnosis: Powerlessness related to ventilator therapy dependency

Immediate Goal(s):

Intermediate Goal(s):

Long-Term Goal(s):

Nursing Interventions   **Expected Outcomes**

ETHICAL QUESTION: CAN PATIENTS REFUSE MECHANICAL VENTILATION?

Discussion:
Mechanical ventilation is a life-support treatment that can be used in a variety of clinical settings including short or long term use for a variety of acute and chronic conditions. Can patients refuse a life support treatment that is keeping them alive? If the withdrawal of the ventilator results in the death of the patient, is the health care worker who removed the ventilator guilty of killing the patient? Can patients refuse mechanical ventilation even if their prognosis with continued treatment is favorable?

Dilemma:
The patient's right to refuse treatment conflicts with the health care worker's obligation to help the patient (autonomy versus beneficence).

Arguments in FAVOR of withdrawing the ventilator at the patient's request:
In the United States, there is a long legal tradition of individual freedom that supports the individual's right to refuse treatment, even if the withholding or withdrawal of that treatment results in the patient's death. The patient's autonomy is more important than the health care worker's obligation to help the patient. The withdrawal of a ventilator is not the same as killing the patient: when a ventilator is withdrawn and the patient dies, the patient dies of his lung or neurological disease, not from the removal of his ventilator. To force patients to stay on ventilators against their will for indeterminate periods of time for marginal or no gains in their health is cruel.

Implications of choosing this position:
Patients will not be subjected to treatments against their will. Patients may refuse life-sustaining treatment — such as ventilators — even if their prognosis is favorable. Patients may elect to be withdrawn from their ventilators for what many health care providers may consider the wrong reasons. Health care providers may feel responsible and guilty about a patient's death that results from a ventilator withdrawal. The acceptance of ventilator withdrawal as "allowing the patient to die" may lead to other forms of killing becoming more socially acceptable.

Arguments AGAINST withdrawing mechanical ventilation at the patient's request:
Human life is precious and should be preserved at all costs. The withdrawal of life support that results directly in the death of the patient is more like killing the patient than allowing the patient to die. Health care workers should not be forced to participate in killing a patient by withdrawing the life support. Patients who might recover and be able to be weaned from their ventilator should not be allowed to withdraw from their life support prematurely.

Implications of choosing this position:
Health care workers may feel guilty about caring for a suffering patient lingering on prolonged mechanical ventilation. Patients on mechanical ventilation against their will may need to be restrained to prevent their self-extubation. Preventing death is more important than respecting patient autonomy.

Potential compromise:
Allow competent patients the right to refuse treatment at any time and for any reason, but do your utmost to encourage patients to avoid hasty, ill-considered, impulsive and destructive decisions.

Implications of choosing this position:
Does not satisfy the objections of those who are against patient refusal of mechanical ventilation. By granting primacy to patient autonomy over health care workers' beneficence, patients would still be able to refuse treatment for hasty, ill-considered, impulsive and destructive reasons.

Guidelines for the nurse caring for a mechanically ventilated patient who requests to have his ventilator withdrawn:

1. Talk with the patient and explore the reasons why the patient wants the ventilator withdrawn. Is the patient's real reason an issue of patient control, lack of sleep, or difficulties in communication? Consider creative nursing measures and collaborative practice interventions that could alleviate the patient's discomforts. Document the discussion, plan of care, interventions and evaluations.

2. If the patient seems willing, explore the issues of death and dying with him and document the discussion. Obtain psychiatric nurse, chaplain and social work consultations if not already in place and if appropriate.

3. Review the patient's chart to verify diagnosis, course of treatment, current treatment goals, current ventilator settings, current comfort measures and their effectiveness, presence of advance directives and any documentation of the patient's competence to make decisions.

4. Discuss the patient's request with his physician. Encourage the physician and the patient to talk with each other about this sensitive issue. Consider the following options: continue the ventilator treatment and initiate measures to alleviate symptoms (pain, lack of sleep) that the patient finds distressing; continue treatment and reassess the efficacy of the treatment in an agreed-upon period of time; discontinue treatment.

5. If the patient has poor and/or inconsistent reasons for wanting to discontinue treatment, consider a psychiatric consultation to help assess the patient's ability to make decisions. If the patient is deemed to be unable to give informed consent to withdraw life support, consult with the patient's decision-maker named in the advances directives, if any, or with the patient's family. If the patient has no family and no advance directives, initiate proceedings for guardianship.

6. If the patient who is able to give informed consent wants his ventilator withdrawn, consult with the patient's physician. The patient, physician and nurse should be able to agree upon an action plan. If not, the nurse should consult with her supervisor and the bioethics committee to discuss the issues.

Bibliography

Applebome P. Judge Rules Quadriplegic Can be Allowed to End Life. The New York Times. 1989 Sept. 7:A16.

Gardner BP. et. al. Ventilation or Dignified Death for Patients with High Tetraplegia. British Medical Journal. 1985 December 7; 291:1620-1622.

Edwards BS. When the Physician Won't Give Up. Am J of Nurs 1993 September; 93(9):34-37.

Maynard FM. The Choice to End Life as a Ventilator-Dependent Quadriplegic. Archives of Physical Medicine and Rehabilitation. 1987 December;68:862-864.

Meisel A. Legal Myths about Terminating Life Support. Archives of Internal Medicine. 1991 August; 151:1497-1501.

Ruark JE. et. al. Initiating and Withdrawing Life Support: Principles and Practice in Adult Medicine. New England Journal of Medicine. 1988 January 7; 318(1):25-30.

ETHICAL QUESTION: SHOULD TERMINAL PATIENTS BE SEDATED BEFORE THEIR VENTILATOR IS WITHDRAWN?

Discussion:

Patients have an ethical and legal right to refuse medical treatment including mechanical ventilation. However, if a patient is awake and alert and extremely dependent on the ventilator, the withdrawal of the ventilator can cause extreme discomfort and distress as the patient experiences air hunger and symptoms of suffocation. Sedation effective enough to alleviate these symptoms can also virtually guarantee that the patient will not survive the ventilator's withdrawal. Should patients be sedated for comfort before ventilator withdrawal, or does such an action effectively constitute killing the patient?

Dilemma:

The obligation to make the patient comfortable for a distressing procedure conflicts with the health care providers' obligation not to harm the patient (beneficence versus non-maleficence). Or, the patient's request for sedation may conflict the obligation not to harm the patient (autonomy versus non-maleficence).

Arguments in FAVOR of sedation before terminal ventilator withdrawal:

Health care providers have an obligation to anticipate distressing symptoms and provide medication to prevent the patient from suffering. The obligation to make the patient comfortable is more important than the provider's fear of harming the patient. It would be cruel not to sedate patients who might experience severe symptoms. Patients for whom ventilator withdrawal symptoms would be severe would probably not survive the ventilator withdrawal. The patient who dies after sedation and ventilator withdrawal dies of his own lung or neurological disease, not from the sedation and the ventilator withdrawal. Ventilator withdrawal allows the patient to die of his own disease; sedation helps to keep him comfortable. Sedation and ventilator withdrawal is not the same as killing the patient.

Implications of choosing this position:

Patients will be sedated at the time of death. Health care workers may feel guilty that they contributed to the patient's death by sedating him. Sedation may contribute to the patient's death or to the time of death. Patients will not experience distressing symptoms of air hunger and suffocation when their ventilators are withdrawn. Patients who might survive their ventilator withdrawal are more likely to die if given sedation.

Arguments AGAINST sedation before terminal ventilator withdrawal:

Sedation before ventilator withdrawal is more like killing the patient than allowing him to die because the sedation will prevent the patient from breathing electively. Health care providers should not be required to assist in what may cause a patient's death. Sedation can be given to a patient after the ventilator is withdrawn if and only if distressing withdrawal symptoms develop.

Implications of choosing this position:

Patients may experience distressing symptoms when their ventilator is withdrawn. Health care professionals may feel guilty if the patient dies after suffering through symptoms of air hunger and suffocation. Patients will be more likely to be able to talk and converse without sedation. Patients who expire without sedation after their ventilators are withdrawn are certain to have died because of their disease process and not from any sedation. Patients who might survive their ventilator withdrawal are more likely to survive without sedation. Sedation given after distressing symptoms occur may be less likely to provide relief.

Potential compromise:

Provide sedation only for those patients considered likely to experience severe withdrawal symptoms. Discuss the pros and cons of sedation with the patient and family and arrive at a joint decision.

Implications of choosing this position:

Health care professionals may still feel that the sedation caused the patient's death. The patient may decide against sedation and suffer distressing symptoms. The patient and family will know what to expect after the ventilator is withdrawn.

Guidelines for the nurse involved in the ventilator withdrawal of a terminally ill patient:

1. Assess if the patient has made an informed choice for the ventilator withdrawal. If you believe that the patient has not made an informed consent, discuss this with the physician and supervisor and consult with the bioethics committee.

2. Assess the patient's reliance on the ventilator by reviewing the chart for the patient's disease process, course of treatment and goals for treatment. Determine the amount of support that the patient receives from the ventilator. In your clinical judgment, is the patient likely to experience symptoms of air hunger and suffocation once the ventilator is removed?

3. If you believe the patient might suffer distressing symptoms upon removal of the ventilator, discuss the issue of sedation with the physician. Develop a plan with the physician for handling the symptoms.

4. Have the physician discuss the issue of sedation with the patient. All persons involved should agree to a plan of care. If a plan of care is not agreed upon, consult with your supervisor and consider a bioethics committee consultation.

5. If the nurse agrees to the plan of care but feels uncomfortable in giving the prescribed sedation, she should inform the physician and ask the physician or another nurse to administer the sedation.

Bibliography

Devettere RJ. Sedation before Ventilator Withdrawal: Can it be Justified by Double Effect and Called "Allowing a Patient to Die"? Journal of Clinical Ethics. 1991 Summer; 2(2):122-125.

Edwards BS and Ueno W. Sedation before Ventilator Withdrawal. Journal of Clinical Ethics. 1991 Summer; 2(2):118-122.

Schneiderman LJ and Spragg RG. Ethical Issues in Discontinuing Mechanical Ventilation. New England Journal of Medicine. 1988 April 14; 318(15): 984-988.

Schneiderman LJ. Is it Morally Justifiable Not to Sedate this Patient before Ventilator Withdrawal? Journal of Clinical Ethics. 1991 Summer; 2(2):129-130.

Wilson WC. et. al. Ordering and Administration of Sedatives and Analgesics During the Withholding and Withdrawal of Life Support from Critically Ill Patients. Journal of the American Medical Association. 1992 February 19; 267(7):949-953.

Truog RD. et. al. Sedation Before Ventilator Withdrawal: Medical and Ethical Considerations. Journal of Clinical Ethics. 1991 Summer; 2(2): 127-129.

Instructional Improvement Tool for Unit

Student feedback/evaluation indicated that I need to improve my classroom presentation by:

Adding Content

1. _____

2. _____

3. _____

Deleting Content

1. _____

2. _____

3. _____

Emphasizing/De-emphasizing the Following Content

1. _____

2. _____

3. _____

Questions students asked that I need to research for the future are:

1. _____

2. _____

3. _____

26
Assessment of Cardiovascular Function

I. Learning Objectives:

In addition to the learning objectives on page 587, I want my students to be able to:

1. _____

2. _____

3. _____

II. Top Terms:

1. Atrioventricular Node
2. Cheyne-Stoke Respirations
3. Crackles
4. Depolarization
5. Friction Rub

6. Gallop Sound
7. Murmurs
8. PMI
9. Sinoatrial Node
10. Wheezes

III. Collaborative Learning Activities:

Team Discussion Questions/Seminar Topics

1. Have students explain why it is important to assess the apical pulse. Identify on each other the two anatomical areas that must be palpated to accurately identify the location of the apex of the heart. (reference pages 601-602)

2. Have students work in four teams. Have each team take one of the four cardiac sounds (gallops, friction rub, murmurs, and clicks/snaps) and compare and contrast each sound relative to timing, intensity, duration, and radiation. What does each sound mean? (reference pages 602-604)

IV. Critical Thinking Activities:

In-Class Team Exercises

Have students compare and contrast the differences in chest pain found with pericarditis, pulmonary pain, and esophageal pain. Use Table 26-1 as a guideline.

	Pain character, location, duration, and radiation	Precipitating Events	Nursing Measures
Pericarditis			
Pain of Pulmonary Origin			
Esophageal Pain			

Send-Home Assignments

Read the following case study. Circle the correct answer.

Case Study: Cardiac Assessment for Chest Pain

Mr. Anderson is a 45-year-old executive with a major oil firm. Lately he has experienced frequent episodes of chest pressure that are relieved with rest. He has requested a complete physical examination. The nurse is to assist with the cardiac assessment. (reference pages 597-600)

1. The nurse takes a baseline blood pressure measurement after the patient has rested for 10 minutes in a supine position. The reading that reflects a reduced pulse pressure is:

    a. 140/90.

    b. 140/100.

    c. 140/110.

    d. 140/120.

2. Five minutes after the initial blood pressure measurement was taken, the nurse assesses additional readings with the patient in a sitting and then a standing position. The reading indicative of an abnormal postural response would be:

    a. lying, 140/110; sitting, 130/100; standing, 135/106.

    b. lying, 140/110; sitting, 135/112; standing, 130/115.

    c. lying, 140/110; sitting, 130/100; standing, 120/90.

    d. lying, 140/110; sitting, 130/108; standing, 125/108.

3. The nurse returns Mr. Anderson to the supine position and measures for jugular vein distention. The finding that would initially indicate an abnormal increase in the volume of the venous system would be obvious distention of the veins with the patient at:

    a. 15 degrees.

    b. 25 degrees.

    c. 35 degrees.

    d. 45 degrees.

27

Management of Patients with Dysrhythmias and Conduction Problems

I. Learning Objectives:

In addition to the learning objectives on page 615, I want my students to be able to:

1. _____

2. _____

3. _____

II. Top Terms:

1. Bigeminy
2. Cardioversion
3. Chronotropic
4. Chryoablation
5. Defibrillation
6. Dysrhythmia
7. Fibrillation
8. Pacemaker
9. Purkinje Network
10. QRS Complex
11. Refractory Period
12. Repolarization

III. Collaborative Learning Activities:

Team Discussion Questions/Seminar Topics

1. Have students explain the differences and related significance between atrial and ventricular dysrhythmias.

2. Have students distinguish between the procedure and nursing implications for cardioversion and defibrillation.

3. Group students into three teams. Have each team present the actions, side-effects, and nursing interventions for use of beta-blockers, channel blockers, and parasympathetic agonists.

IV. Critical Thinking Activities:

In-Class Team Exercises

1. Review these four ECG rhythm strips. Identify the dysrhythmia in each and discuss, as a group, the associated symptomatology, medical and nursing interventions. (reference pages 620-624)

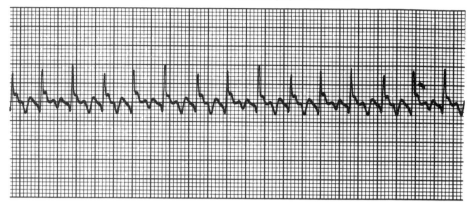

Figure 27-9

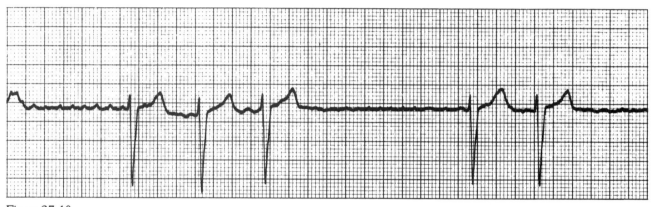

Figure 27-10

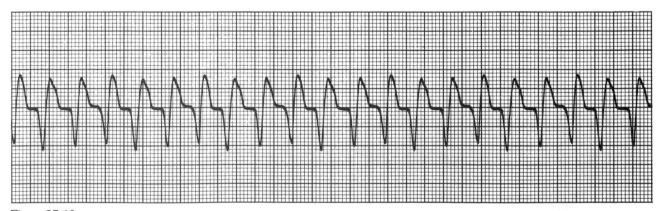

Figure 27-13

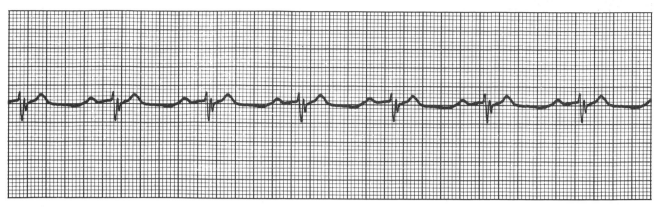

Figure 27-15

2. For each of these pathophysiological responses, have students graphically illustrate a dysthrythmia that reflects the altered cardiac functioning. (reference pages 618-619, Figure 27-4)

    A. Cardiac tissue ischemia

    B. Cardiac muscle injury

    C. Infarcted tissue

IV. Critical Thinking Activities:

Send Home Assignments

1. Draw on a graphic sheet the depolarization-repolarization sequence that illustrates the electrical conduction system of the heart.

2. Read the following case study. Fill in the blanks or circle the correct answer.

Case Study: Permanent Pacemaker

Mr. Wilkens is a 58-year-old Asian male who is scheduled for permanent pacemaker insertion as treatment for a tachydysrhythmia that doesn't respond to medication therapy. He will have an endocardial implant. Answer the following questions based upon your knowledge of pacemaker management. (reference pages 629-633)

1. Mr. Wilkens' pacemaker is set at 72 beats/min. His heart rate is 76. Is this expected? (Yes/No) Explain the rationale for your answer.

2. Nursing care includes incision site assessment for three complications: a. _____,
   b. _____, and c. _____.

3. The *most common* postoperative complication is _____ which can be prevented by
   _____.

4. List six (6) things about the pacemaker that must be noted on a patient's chart:

   a. _____   d. _____

   b. _____   e. _____

   c. _____   f. _____

5. Describe nursing interventions and expected outcomes that should be used to meet the three (3) major goals of patient care.

Goals	Nursing Activities	Expected Outcomes
a. _____	a. _____	a. _____
b. _____	b. _____	b. _____
c. _____	c. _____	c. _____

6. Explain what assessment criteria will be used to determine if expected outcomes of care are achieved.

Expected Outcomes	Assessment Criteria
a. Freedom from Infection	_____
b. Adherence to a Self-Care Program	_____
c. Maintenance of Pacemaker Function	_____

28

Management of Patients with Cardiac Disorders and Related Complications

I. Learning Objectives:

In addition to the learning objectives on page 637, I want my students to be able to:

1. _____

2. _____

3. _____

II. Top Terms:

1. Afterload
2. Angina Pectoris
3. Atheroma
4. Atheroscleratic Coronary Heart Disease
5. Cardiac Output (CO = HR x SV)
6. Cardiac Tamponade
7. Coronary Artery Bypass Graft Surgery (CABG)
8. Coronary Artery Revascularization

9. Myocardial Infarction
10. Pericardial Effusion
11. Percutaneous Transluminal Coronary Angioplasty (PTCA)
12. Preload
13. Prinzmetal's Angina
14. Streptokinase
15. Stroke Volume

III. Collaborative Learning Activities:

Team Discussion Questions/Seminar Topics

1. Have students divide into two teams. Have each team compare and contrast the etiology, clinical manifestations, diagnostic evaluation, medical management, and nursing interventions for a patient with angina pectoris and one with a myocardial infarction. (reference pages 638-654)

2. Have students explain the rationale for modifying specific risk factors associated with heart disease. (reference pages 636-638)

3. Choose a team to present the scientific rationale for a special diet for heart disease along with some of the reasons why dietary management is controversial. (reference pages 639 and 648)

IV. Critical Thinking Exercises:

In-Class Team Exercises

1. Discuss the formation of atheromatous plaques in an artery, using the following terms in your explanation: *atheroma*, *blood clots*, *lumen*, and *tunica intima*.

2. For each of the drug classifications commonly used to treat angina pectoris, outline specific actions, rationales, and associated nursing implications.

	Action	Rationale	Nursing Implications
Nitrates			
Beta-adrenergic Blockers			
Calcium Ion Antagonists			

Send-Home Assignments

Compare and contrast the purpose and function of an intracoronary artery stent (Figure 28-4) and a shunt catheter (Figure 28-5). Develop a preoperative and postoperative nursing care plan for a 47-year-old male who would be receiving either treatment.

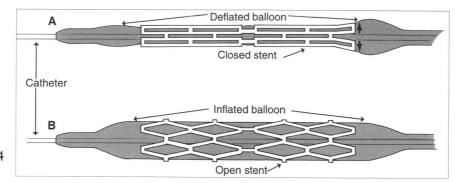

Figure 28-4

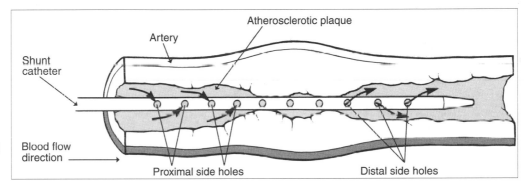

Figure 28-5

Read the following case studies. Fill in the blanks or circle the correct answer.

Case Study: Pulmonary Edema

Mr. Wolman is to be discharged from the hospital to home. He is 79 years old, lives with his wife, and has just recovered from mild pulmonary edema secondary to congestive heart failure. (reference pages 654-661)

1. The most common cause of pulmonary edema is _____.

2. You know that the sequence of pathophysiological events are triggered by:

   a. elevated left ventricular end-diastolic pressure.

   b. elevated pulmonary venous pressure.

   c. increased hydrostatic pressure.

   d. impaired lymphatic drainage.

3. The nurse advises Mr. Wolman to rest frequently at home. Her advice is based on the knowledge that rest:

   a. decreases blood pressure.

   b. increases the heart reserve.

   c. reduces the work of the heart.

   d. does all of the above.

4. The nurse reminds Mr. Wolman to sleep with two pillows to elevate his head about 10 inches. This position is recommended because:

   a. preload can be increased, thus enhancing cardiac output.

   b. pulmonary congestion can be reduced.

   c. venous return to the lungs can be improved, thus reducing peripheral edema.

   d. all of the above can help relieve his symptoms.

5. Mr. Wolman takes 0.25 mg of digoxin once a day. The nurse should tell him about signs of digitalis toxicity, which include:

   a. anorexia.

   b. bradycardia and tachycardia.

   c. nausea and vomiting.

   d. all of the above.

6. Mr. Wolman also takes Lasix (40 mg) twice a day. He is aware of signs related to hypokalemia and supplements his diet with foods high in potassium, such as:

   a. bananas.

   b. raisins.

   c. orange juice.

   d. all of the above.

ETHICAL QUESTION: WHEN IS IT APPROPRIATE TO CONSIDER WITHHOLDING OR WITHDRAWING LIFE SUPPORT?

Discussion: Life support can include an intra-aortic balloon pump, ventilators, vasoactive infusions, CPR, and antibiotics. Patients receiving these treatments include acutely, chronically and terminally ill patients. Often, when dependent on life-support, a patient may be unable to make decisions about his own care and the family may be in crisis. At what point is it appropriate to raise the delicate issue of withholding or withdrawing life support?

Dilemma: The patient's right to choose or refuse treatment conflicts with the obligation to do what is best for the patient (autonomy versus beneficence). Or, the patient's right to choose or refuse treatment conflicts with the obligation not to harm the patient with threatening or inappropriate questions at the wrong time (autonomy versus non-maleficence).

Arguments that discussions about the limitations of life-supporting treatment should be held when patients are admitted to the hospital: All patients would have the opportunity to discuss the possible treatment options open to them and to express their opinions and reservations about different treatment goals and therapeutic measures. Formalized requirements to have such discussions on admission would ensure that patients' treatment preferences would be addressed and documented.

Implications of choosing this position: Not all patients are able to maintain a coherent and detailed discussion on admission (such as those who are confused or comatose on admission). Patients who are admitted to the hospital in relatively good health (such as for childbirth or elective surgery) may express treatment preferences that might conflict with those that they would choose if they became critically ill. Patients might experience circumstances (such as life-supporting treatment) differently than they had anticipated. Some patients who are acutely ill at admission may find a discussion about limiting life support threatening, frightening and inappropriate.

Arguments that discussions about the limitations of life-supporting treatment should be done only when certain circumstances arise: Patients are deemed to have consented to treatment to sustain life unless certain circumstances occur that would cause either the patient or the care givers to question if life support should be withheld or withdrawn. Some widely supported circumstances under which discussions of limiting life-supporting should occur are (1) when the patient's death is imminent; (2) When a cardiac or respiratory arrest is anticipated and the patient is either unlikely to survive resuscitation or it is likely that if he survives he will suffer a poor outcome, such as neurological impairment; (3) when life supporting treatment is not or is unlikely to achieve the treatment goals for the patient; (4) when the patient's suffering; or (5) when the patient raises questions about the appropriateness of treatment.

Implications of choosing this position: The timing of discussions is crucial; use of the above criteria may result in delay of discussion until the patient has deteriorated too far and is no longer able to express his preferences about treatment. Patients may suffer greatly before discussions about withholding or withdrawing life support treatment are initiated.

Potential compromise: Maintain open lines of communication with all patients about their treatment goals and preferences before hospital admission and throughout the hospital stay. Each conversation with the patient about treatment goals and preferences should be documented.

Implications of choosing this option: All patients will have the opportunity to discuss their treatment preferences under varied and changing circumstances. Discussions can be timed to occur at appropriate times for the patient. Staff work requirements will be increased when patients require numerous detailed discussions.

Role of the nurse in discussion about the withholding or withdrawing of life-support:

1. Familiarize yourself with all aspects of the patient's case. Review the chart for the patient's history, reason for admission, course of treatment, treatment goals, documentation of previous discussions about limiting treatment, and the existence of any advances directives.

2. Be present for all discussions between the patient and the physician.

3. Act as a patient advocate during discussions about treatment choices. Encourage the patient to speak up and ask questions or state his desires about treatment. Document all conversations about treatment preferences.

4. Facilitate a patient care conference if necessary to enhance communication and resolve a disagreement about withholding and withdrawing life support.

5. If a patient care conference fails to produce an agreement about a plan of care, inform your supervisor and consult with the bioethics committee.

6. Use your nursing judgment about the patient's condition to plan the urgency and timing of the above interventions.

Bibliography

Abrams FR.   Withholding Treatment When Death is Not Imminent. Geriatrics. 1987 May; 42(5): 77-84.

Battin MP. The Least Worst Death. Hastings Center Report. 1983 April; 13(2): 13-16.

Iwersen E. Life at What Cost? Am J of Nurs. 1988 May; 88(5): 639.

Meisel A. Legal Myths about Terminating Life Support. Archives of Internal Medicine. 1991 August; 151: 1497-1502.

Ruark JE and Raffin TA. Initiating and Withdrawing Life Support: Principles and Practice in Adult Medicine. New England Journal of Medicine. 1988 January 7; 318(l): 25-30.

Tomlinson T and Brody H. Ethics and Communication in Do-Not-Resuscitate Orders. New England Journal of Medicine. 1988 January 7; 318(l): 43-46.

Zugar A. High Hopes. Journal of the American Medical Association. 1989 December 1; 262(21): 2988.

ETHICAL QUESTION: WHAT DOES DNR MEAN?

Discussion:

At the time of its inception in the early 1960's, CPR was intended only for patients with unexpected cardiac arrest who stood a good chance for recovery. Thirty years later, all patients admitted to a hospital are deemed to have consented to full resuscitation measures unless a Do Not Resuscitate (DNR) order has been written for the patient. DNR orders are most often written for critically ill or terminally ill patients. Does the DNR order therefore refer only to actions concerning cardiac or respiratory arrest, or does a DNR order imply that a non-aggressive care plan has been instituted for a patient? Patients, physicians and nurses may have different ideas about what DNR means, ranging from "do not start CPR" to "keep the patient comfortable" to "do not notify MD of abnormal laboratory results" to "do not admit to the ICU."

Dilemma:

The patient and various practitioners have different ideas about what the DNR order means and what is best for the patient (beneficence versus beneficence).

Arguments that a DNR order is the SAME THING as a non-aggressive care plan:

DNR orders are most often written for critically ill and terminally ill patients. If such patients would not survive a cardiac or respiratory arrest or would not want resuscitation measures performed, then they probably would not want other invasive, aggressive treatment as well (such as vasopressors or an intra-aortic balloon pump). Keeping someone comfortable does not include invasive, aggressive measures.

Implications of choosing this position:

There will be confusion among caregivers as to what interventions are and are not required. For example, is dopamine prescribed for the purpose of promoting renal perfusion considered to be aggressive therapy? Patients might not receive interventions that might benefit them if these are considered aggressive. Physicians might avoid writing DNR orders for fear that appropriate interventions would not be initiated for their patients and that nurses would not notify them of acute changes in their patient's condition.

Arguments that a DNR order is NOT the same thing as a nonaggressive care plan:

A DNR order does not address any other situations other than a cardiac or respiratory arrest. To imply that it does creates confusion. DNR patients can appropriately receive high-tech life supportive measures and aggressive treatment for symptomatic control (such as a ventilator for shortness of breath) or to treat the underlying disease (chemotherapy to treat a tumor). The aggressiveness or non-aggressiveness of the pain of care can be addressed outside of the DNR order. DNR orders are appropriate for different patients for different reasons. Not all DNR patients are alike.

Implications of choosing this position:

There is less confusion about treatment that is covered and not covered by the order. Some patients may be treated more aggressively than they may desire.

Potential compromise:

Decisions about DNR status should also include decisions about how to handle other acute patient changes, for example: "DNR — for shortness of breath page MD stat" or, "DNR —notify MD for systolic blood pressure less than 100," or "DNR — keep patient comfortable, use morphine as prescribed.

Implications of choosing this position:

There will be less confusion about what is required for patient care. The discussion and decisions required for a simple DNR order will be more complicated and time consuming. Physicians may avoid writing DNR orders if too many other decisions are required at the same time.

Guidelines for the nurse caring for a patient whose status is DNR:

1. Verify DNR status by checking the chart for the original order.

2. Review the chart for the patient's history, reason for admission, course of treatment, current care plan and treatment goals. Distinguish DNR order from care plan and treatment goals of the patient. Assure yourself that the DNR order is in accordance with the patient's wishes and the patient's condition.

3. If, in your nursing judgment, you anticipate a deterioration in the patient's condition, notify the physician and discuss the plan of care for the patient, including specifics as to what patient conditions (e.g., changes in lab values or vital signs) the physician does and does not want to act upon. Document this information in the nurses' notes and on the physician order sheet. Communicate this information accurately at the change of shift.

4. Assure the patient and the physician that you will provide the patient with expert and vigilant nursing care.

5. In the absence of a well-documented plan to the contrary, inform the physician of all acute changes in the patient's condition just as you would for any other patient.

6. As death approaches for a patient with a non-aggressive care plan, use nursing interventions to promote patient comfort. Consult with the physician as appropriate for medical interventions that may help to provide comfort. Provide emotional support for the patient and the family. Allow the family liberal visiting privileges. Provide for privacy as possible. Consider chaplaincy support as appropriate.

Bibliography

Council on Ethical and Judicial Affairs, American Medical Association. Guidelines for the Appropriate Use of DNR Orders. Journal of the American Medical Association. 1991 April 10; 265(.14): 1868-1875.

Edwards BS. Does the DNR Patient Belong in the ICU? Crit Care Nurs Clin North Am. 1990 September; 2(3): 473-480.

The Hastings Center. Guidelines of the Termination of Life-Sustaining Treatment and the Care of the Dying. Briarcliff Manor, N.Y., The Hastings Center, 1987: 48-52.

Lipton HL. Do-Not-Resuscitate Decisions in a Community Hospital: Incidence, Implications and Outcomes. Journal of the American Medical Association. 1986 September 5; 256(9): 1164- 1169.

Martin DA and Redland AR. Legal and Ethical Issues in Resuscitation and Withholding of Treatment. Crit Care Nurse Quarterly. 1988 March; 10(4): 1-8.

Nolan K. In Death's Shadow: The Meanings of Withholding Resuscitation. Hastings Center Report. 1987 October-November; 17(5): 9-14.

Sulmasy DP. et. al. The Quality of Mercy: Caring for Patients with

Do-Not-Resuscitate Orders. Journal of the American Medical Association. 1992 February 5; 267(5): 682-686.

Youngner SJ. et. al. "Do Not Resuscitate Orders": Incidence and Implications in a Medical Intensive Care Unit. Journal of the American Medical Association. 1985 January 4; 253(l): 54- 57.

Youngner SJ. Do Not Resuscitate Orders: No Longer a Secret But Still a Problem. Hastings Center Report. 1987 February; 17(l): 2433.

29

Management of Patients with Structural, Infectious, or Inflammatory Cardiac Disorders

I. Learning Objectives:

In addition to the learning objectives on page 677, I want my students to be able to:

1. _____

2. _____

3. _____

II. Top Terms:

1. Cardiomyopathy
2. Chordoplasty
3. Commissurotomy
4. Endocarditis
5. Mitral Valve Prolapse

6. Myocarditis
7. Osler Nodes
8. Valvuloplasty
9. Vegetations

III. Collaborative Learning Activities:

Team Discussion Questions/Seminar Topics

1. Have students compare and contrast infective endocarditis to rheumatic endocarditis relative to pathophysiology, clinical manifestations, nursing and medical management and prevention.

2. Have students discuss the nursing care activities for patients with congestive, hypertrophic and restrictive cardiomyopathies.

IV. Critical Thinking Activities:

In-Class Team Exercises

1. Complete the following chart comparing the valvular disorders of the heart. (reference pages 678-680)

	Pathophysiology	Clinical Manifestations	Management	Nursing Interventions
MITRAL VALVES				
Prolapse				
Stenosis				
Insufficiency				
AORTIC VALVE				
Stenosis				
Insufficiency				

2. Examine Figure 29-2. Describe in detail the procedure commonly used in mitral and aortic valve stenosis including implications for nursing care activities. (reference pages 680-682)

Send-Home Assignments

Draft a nursing care plan for preoperative and postoperative nursing interventions for a patient undergoing valvuloplasty. (reference pages 680-682)

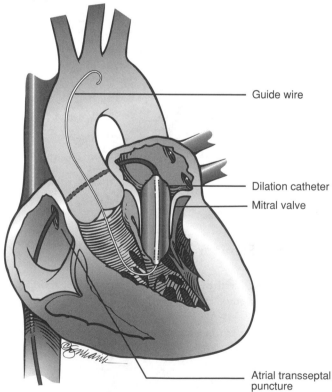

Guide wire

Dilation catheter

Mitral valve

Atrial transseptal puncture

Figure 29-2

Read the following case study. Fill in the blanks or circle the correct answer.

Case Study: Acute Pericarditis

Mrs. Russell is a 46-year-old Caucasian who developed symptoms of acute pericarditis secondary to a viral infection. Diagnosis was based on the characteristic sign of a friction rub and pain over the pericardium. (reference pages 690-692)

1. Based on your knowledge of pericardial pain, you suggest the following body position to relieve the pain symptoms:

    a. flat in bed with feet slightly higher than the head

    b. Fowler's

    c. right side-lying

    d. semi-Fowler's

2. Based on assessment data, choose the major nursing diagnosis: _____

3. Initial nursing intervention includes maintenance of bed rest until the following symptom(s) disappear:

    a. fever

    b. friction rub

    c. pain

    d. all of the above

4. Identify three drug classifications that are commonly prescribed for management/treatment:

    a.

    b.

    c.

5. Draw the chest wall and name the anatomical landmarks used to auscultate for a pericardial friction rub.

6. List the two major expected patient outcomes for nursing management of a patient with pericarditis.

    a.

    b.

30

Management of the Cardiac Surgery Patient

I. Learning Objectives:

In addition to the learning objectives on page 695, I want my students to be able to:

1. _____

2. _____

3. _____

II. Top Terms:

1. Afterload
2. Anxiolytic Medication
3. Centrifugal Pumps
4. Coagulopathies

5. Cyclosporine
6. Extracorporeal Circulation
7. Preload
8. Postcardiotomy Psychosis

III. Collaborative Learning Activities:

Team Discussion Questions/Seminar Topics

1. Have students explain the altered blood flow for a patient on a cardiopulmonary bypass machine.

2. Ask the students to distinguish between the two types of heart transplants, the orthotopic and heterotopic procedures. List specific pre and postoperative nursing interventions for each procedure.

IV. Critical Thinking Activities:

In-Class Team Exercises

1. Have students develop a nursing care plan for a patient who will be undergoing cardiac surgery. Have each team take one nursing diagnosis and examine it related to nursing interventions, rationale, and expected outcomes. Use the Nursing Care Plan on pages 708-714 as a guide.

2. Assign groups of students to research the latest developments in the use of artificial hearts beginning with the Jarvik-7. Have them use articles from medical and nursing journals and argue for and against the use of such hearts for patients of varying age ranges.

Case Study: Coronary Artery Bypass Graft Surgery

Mrs. Connor, a 63-year-old retired businesswoman, has just undergone coronary artery bypass graft (CABG) surgery. A portion of her saphenous vein was used for the graft. (reference pages 696-707)

1. Immediate postoperative nursing actions for Mrs. Connor include:

    a. change of body position every 1 to 2 hours after her condition stabilizes.

    b. deep breathing and coughing to open alveolar sacs and increase perfusion.

    c. suctioning to remove secretions from the endotracheal tube.

    d. all of the above.

2. Postoperative early extubation is considered when:

    a. blood gas determinations are adequate.

    b. pressures are within 20% of preoperative volumes.

    c. tidal volume is sufficient.

    d. all of the above occur.

3. Mrs. Connor's kidney function is evaluated as an indicator of cardiac output. Inadequate cardiac output is reflected by:

    a. a decreased urine osmolality.

    b. an hourly urine output of 60 ml.

    c. a specific gravity of 1.032.

    d. all of the above.

4. Several days postoperatively Mrs. Connor exhibits tingling in her toes, carpopedal spasm, and tetany. The nurse knows that these symptoms are associated with:

    a. hypercalcemia.

    b. hypernatremia.

    c. hypocalcemia.

    d. hypokalemia.

31

Assessment and Management of Patients with Vascular Disorders and Problems of Peripheral Circulation

I. Learning Objectives:

In addition to the learning objectives on page 719, I want my students to be able to:

1. _____

2. _____

3. _____

II. Top Terms:

1. Buerger-Allen Exercises
2. Capacitance Vessels
3. Doppler Ultrasonography
4. Essential Hypertension
5. Fusiform Aneurysm

6. Homan's Sign
7. Intermittent Claudication
8. Ischemia
9. Phlebothrombosis
10. Thrombophlebitis

III. Collaborative Learning Activities:

Team Discussion Questions/Seminar Topics

1. Divide the class into two groups and have the students compare and contrast the differences in alterations in blood flow in veins, arteries, and lymph vessels.

2. Have a group of students present opposing theories of the pathogenesis of atherosclerosis and have each team defend their theory with scientific facts.

IV. Critical Thinking Activities:

In-Class Team Exercises

1. Draw a capillary and label the arterial and venous ends. The microcirculation between the blood and the interstitial fluid depends on the equilibrium between the hydrostatic and oncotic forces of the blood and the interstitium. Depict the direction of fluid movement and explain the fluid dynamics, using symbols instead of the exact pressures in millimeters of mercury. A supplementary physiology textbook will be needed as a reference if the students wish to label their drawing with exact pressures.

2. Assign a team of students to demonstrate Buerger-Allen exercises and defend their action with scientific rationales.

3. Divide the students into teams. Have them examine the Algorithm in Figure 31-11 in reference to patients with varying blood pressure measurements. Have them modify the algorithm as necessary.

Send-Home Assignments

Have the student complete the following schematic.

Pathophysiology of Essential Hypertension

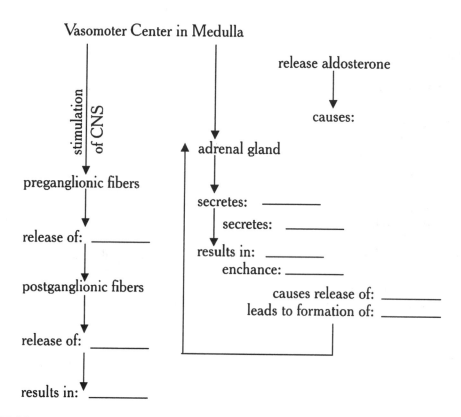

Vasomoter Center in Medulla

stimulation of CNS

release aldosterone

causes:

adrenal gland

preganglionic fibers

secretes: ————

secretes: ————

release of: ————

results in: ————

enchance: ————

postganglionic fibers

causes release of: ————

leads to formation of: ————

release of: ————

results in: ————

Reference   pages 53-54.

Read the following case study. Circle the correct answer.

Case Study: Thrombophlebitis

Hazel seeks medical attention for left calf pain and tenderness, which seems to be relieved with rest. Hazel is 38-years-old and recently delivered her seventh child. (reference pages 752-757)

1. Hazel's medical diagnosis is superficial thrombophlebitis. The nurse knows that Hazel's thrombus development could be associated with the antecedent factors of:

    a. altered blood coagulation.

    b. blood stasis.

    c. vessel wall injury.

    d. all of the above.

2. Clinical manifestations *specific for deep venous thrombosis* that are associated with Hazel's diagnosis include all of the following *except*:

    a. a positive Homan's sign.

    b. local tenderness and induration.

    c. redness and warmth.

    d. swelling and pain in the involved area.

3. Hazel is hospitalized and heparin is started by intermittent infusion. Her daily dose is calculated by measuring the:

    a. circulation time.

    b. partial thromboplastin time.

    c. prothrombin time.

    d. thrombin clotting time.

4. While monitoring Hazel's response to heparinization, the nurse recalls that anticoagulant therapy cannot:

    a. delay the clotting time of the blood.

    b. dissolve a thrombus that has already formed.

    c. forestall the extension of a thrombus once it has formed.

    d. prevent the formation of a thrombus.

5. Nursing measures for heparin administration include making sure that the antagonist to heparin is available, which is:

    a. phytonadione solution or tablets.

    b. pilocarpine nitrate.

    c. promethazine hydrochloride.

    d. protamine sulfate.

32

Assessment and Management of Patients with Hematologic Disorders

I. Learning Objectives:

In addition to the learning objectives on page 767, I want my students to be able to:

1. _____

2. _____

3. _____

II. Top Terms:

1. Agranulocytosis
2. Ecchymosis
3. Erythropoiesis
4. Hematopoietic
5. Hodgkin's Disease

6. Idiopathic
7. Leukopenia
8. Petechiae
9. Polycythemia
10. Thrombocytopenia

III. Collaborative Learning Activities:

Team Discussion Questions/Seminar Topics

1. Have students compare and contrast the etiology, diagnostic evaluation, clinical manifestations, medical management and nursing care for a patient with Hodgkin's disease and one with Leukemia.

2. Assign students to two teams. Have the teams present the differences in treatment approaches to anticoagulation using heparin versus coumadin. Use sample laboratory reports from the clinical area to correlate data.

IV. Critical Thinking Activities:

In-Class Team Exercises

1. Have students explain the purpose and procedure involved in a bone marrow biopsy. Have each student identify the sites on a partner and describe any pre-procedure instructions that should be given.

2. Assign students to two to four work groups and have them complete the following chart comparing the various types of anemia as to etiology, diagnostic evaluation, clinical manifestations, and medical and nursing management.

Type of Anemia	Etiology	Dx Evaluation	Clinical Manifestations	Medical Rx	Nursing Care
Aplastic Anemia					
Anemias in Renal Disease					
Anemias in Chronic Diseases					
Iron-Deficiency Anemia					
Megaloblastic Anemias					
Sickle Cell Anemia					

Send-Home Assignments

Read the following case study. Fill in the blanks or circle the correct answer.

Case Study: Leukemia

John is a 51-year-old accountant recently diagnosed with acute myelogenous leukemia. (reference pages 791-792)

1. Acute myelogenous leukemia affects the _____.

2. A bone marrow specimen is diagnostic if it shows an excess of _____.

3. A characteristic symptom that results from insufficient red blood cell production is:

   a. bleeding tendencies.

   b. fatigue.

   c. susceptibility to infection.

   d. all of the above.

4. Survival rates for those who receive treatment average:

   a. 6 months.

   b. 1 year.

   c. 2 years.

   d. 5 years.

5. The major form of therapy that frequently results in remission is:

   a. bone marrow transplantation.

   b. chemotherapy.

   c. radiation.

   d. surgical intervention.

Instructional Improvement Tool for Unit

Student feedback/evaluation indicated that I need to improve my classroom presentation by:

Adding Content

1. _____
   _____

2. _____
   _____

3. _____
   _____

Deleting Content

1. _____
   _____

2. _____
   _____

3. _____
   _____

Emphasizing/De-emphasizing the Following Content

1. _____
   _____

2. _____
   _____

3. _____
   _____

Questions students asked that I need to research for the future are:

1. _____
   _____

2. _____
   _____

3. _____
   _____

33

Assessment of Digestive and Gastrointestinal Function

I. Learning Objectives:

In addition to the learning objectives on page 815, I want my students to be able to:

1. _____

2. _____

3. _____

II. Top Terms:

1. Ampulla of Vater
2. Detoxification
3. Endoscopy
4. Flatulence
5. Gastric Analysis

6. Hematemesis
7. Intrinsic Factor
8. Manometry
9. Peristalsis
10. Sigmoidoscopy

III. Collaborative Learning Activities:

Team Discussion Questions/Seminar Topics

1. Have students describe the purpose, patient preparation, and procedure for radiographic diagnostic tests on the upper and lower gastrointestinal tract.

2. Ask students to divide into three teams and have each team present the similarities and differences between ultrasonography, computed tomography, and magnetic resonance imaging as they pertain to the examination of the digestive system.

IV. Critical Thinking Activities:

In-Class Team Exercises

1. Divide the students into two teams and have them work with Figure 33-2. Have Team A draw the innervation of the sympathetic and parasympathetic parts of the autonomic system. Have Team B draw the blood supply, paying particular attention to the superior and inferior mesenteric arteries. (reference pages 816-818)

34

Management of Patients with Ingestive Problems and Upper Gastrointestinal Disorders

I. Learning Objectives:

In addition to the learning objectives on page 831, I want my students to be able to:

1. _____

2. _____

3. _____

II. Top Terms:

1. Achalasia
2. Diverticulum
3. Dysphasia
4. Hypoglossal
5. Odynophagia

6. Parotitis
7. Pyrosis
8. Sialolithiasis
9. Stomatitis
10. Xerostomia

III. Collaborative Learning Activities:

Team Discussion Questions/Seminar Topics

1. Assign students the topic, "Abnormalities of the Salivary Glands." Have students compare and contrast the differences and nursing interventions for parotitis, sialadenitis, sialothiasis, and neoplasms of the parotid.

IV. Critical Thinking Activities

In-Class Exercises

1. Dawn is a 23-year-old who has just been examined in the physician's office and diagnosed with herpes simplex on the upper lip. She was given a prescription for Acyclovir. The MD asks you, the nurse, to give her any health teaching information she may need before she leaves. To develop your plan, choose the information heading you believe is significant and then outline a teaching guide. Write a rationale for each action.

    Associated Data:

    -   Dawn has heavy blood flow during her menstrual cycle.
    -   Dawn plans to work as a lifeguard at the shore beginning next month.
    -   She eats out frequently, especially in Mexican and Italian restaurants.
    -   She will be living with three roommates in a small, summer cottage.
    -   She has limited income and is just recovering from infectious mononucleosis.

2. Compare and contrast the symptomatology of a dentoalveolar and periapical abscess. Have students develop a preventive teaching plan for young adults who use a health clinic located on a university campus. Suggest that one or more students illustrate the differences on posters that can be placed on bulletin boards near the health center.

Send-Home Assignments

Read the following case study. Fill in the blanks or circle the correct answer.

Case Study: Cancer of the Mouth

Edith, a 64-year-old mother of two, has been a chain smoker for 20 years. During the past month she noticed a dryness in her mouth and a roughened area that is irritating. She mentioned her symptoms to her dentist, who referred her to a medical internist. (reference pages 837-841)

1. Based on the patient's health history, the nurse suspects oral cancer. Describe what the nurse would expect the lesion to look like.

   _____

2. During the health history the nurse noted that Edith did not mention a late-occurring symptom of mouth cancer, which is:

   a. drainage.

   b. fever.

   c. odor.

   d. pain.

3. On physical examination Edith evidenced changes associated with cancer of the mouth, such as:

   a. a sore, roughened area that has not healed in 3 weeks.

   b. minor swelling in an area adjacent to the lesion.

   c. numbness in the affected area of the mouth.

   d. all of the above.

4. To confirm a diagnosis of carcinoma of the mouth, a physician would order:

   a. a biopsy.

   b. a staining procedure.

   c. exfoliative cytology.

   d. roentgenography.

5. List three therapies that are considered effective for treatment:

   _____

   _____

   _____

6. Edith chose to have the lesion surgically removed. A priority postoperative nursing measure is to:

   a. keep the incisional area as dry as possible.

   b. keep the mouth clean.

   c. maintain an airway.

   d. reduce the number of transient bacteria.

7. Follow-up care for Edith is based on the knowledge that:

   a. chemotherapy is a necessary part of postoperative management and should be continued for 2 to 3 years.

   b. prophylactic radiotherapy is routinely scheduled.

   c. surgical intervention in the early stages of cancer is always curative.

   d. 90% of recurrences will appear within the first 18 months.

35

Gastrointestinal Intubation and Special Nutritional Management

I. Learning Objectives:

In addition to the learning objectives on page 857, I want my students to be able to:

1. _____

2. _____

3. _____

II. Top Terms:

1. Decompression
2. Dumping Syndrome
3. Gastrostomy
4. Hyperalimentation
5. Negative Nitrogen Balance
6. PEG catheter
7. Total Nutrient Admixture

III. Collaborative Learning Activities:

Team Discussion Questions/Seminar Topics

1. Have students outline and discuss the specific method for determining nasogastric tube placement. Discuss the research findings of Metheny, et al (1993) regarding accurate assessment of tube placement.

2. Discuss why the dumping syndrome occurs and what nursing measures can be used to prevent its occurrence.

3. Design a nursing care plan for a patient with a gastrostomy tube. Based on the six nursing diagnoses listed on page 871, have six groups of students each design one component of the plan of care. Challenge the students to *cluster related data* to support their plan.

IV. Critical Thinking Exercises

In-Class Team Exercises

1. Bring several nasogastric and/or nasoenteric tubes to class. Based on the purposes of intubation (decompression, diagnosis, medication administration/feeding, treatment for obstruction or bleeding, or specimen collection) have students *determine specific nursing interventions* for teaching patients about insertion and management.

2. Ask students to develop a patient teaching guide for a patient for home administration of an enteral feeding. Allow students to choose the patient profile (age, socioeconomic status, financial status) they want to use.

3. Have a group of students draw a PEG catheter on sheet paper or the blackboard. Ask members of the group to explain the scientific rationale for tube placement and the use of various parts/components; e.g., the external cross-bar.

Send-Home Assignments

Read the following case study. Circle the correct answer.

Case Study: Total Parenteral Nutrition

Penny is 30-years-old and single. She is 5 feet 7 inches tall, weighs 150 pounds, and is receiving total parenteral nutrition solution at the rate of 3 liters per day. Her postoperative condition warrants her receiving nutrients by the intravenous route. (reference pages 874-879)

1. The nurse knows that to spare body protein, Penny's daily calorie intake must be:

    a. about 500 calories per day.

    b. approximately 1500 calories per day.

    c. around 800 calories per day.

    d. equal to 1000 calories per day.

2. The nurse estimates Penny's caloric intake for each 1000 ml of total parenteral nutrition to yield a glucose concentration of:

    a. 500 calories.

    b. 800 calories.

    c. 1000 calories

    d. 1500 calories.

3. Penny's parenteral nutrition infusion rate is 120 ml/hr. Her rate has slowed because of positional body changes. To compensate, the nurse could safely increase Penny's rate for 8 hours to:

    a. 100 ml/hr.

    b. 125 ml/hr.

    c. 138 ml/hr.

    d. 146 ml/hr.

4. The nurse should observe Penny for signs of rapid fluid intake, which may include:

    a. chills.

    b. fever.

    c. nausea.

    d. all of the above.

5. The nurse weighs Penny daily. After 7 days, Penny's weight gain is abnormal at:

    a.   3.5 pounds.

    b.   5 pounds.

    c.   7 pounds.

    d.   12 pounds.

ETHICAL QUESTION: IS IT PERMISSIBLE TO WITHHOLD OR WITHDRAW NUTRITION AND HYDRATION FROM PATIENTS WHO CANNOT EAT OR DRINK?

Discussion:

It is generally agreed that patients (or their designated decision-makers) can refuse life saving treatment. Nutrition and hydration, however, are perceived as food and drink because they can be provided often by low-tech means and because withdrawing or withholding them can result in the patient becoming dehydrated or even literally starving to death. Thus, some have argued that nutrition and hydration should always to be provided to every patient, regardless of the patient's preferences or the patient's condition.

Dilemma:

The patient's desire to have nutrition or hydration withdrawn or withheld conflicts with others' reluctance not to harm the patient by withdrawing the food and water needed for survival (autonomy versus non-maleficence).

Arguments AGAINST the withholding and withdrawing of nutrition and hydration:

Nutrition and hydration — however administered — are symbolic of food and drink, and like nursing care, should be provided for every patient. Nutrition and hydration are relatively easy to provide with low-tech means. The withholding or withdrawing of nutrition and hydration is more like killing the patient than allowing the patient to die of his, own disease because when nutrition and hydration are withdrawn, the patient will definitely die of starvation and dehydration, not of the underlying disease.

Implications of choosing this position:

Chronically and terminally ill patients will live longer in perhaps a debilitated state. Health care costs will rise due to the long term care of these patients. Debilitated patients being maintained on nutrition and hydration may be seen as a factor in the high costs of health care. Restraints may be needed to maintain feeding in some patients. The provision of nutrition and hydration has side effects that may prove distressing to the patient (such as diarrhea or infection). The provision of nutrition and hydration becomes a special category of life support. Criteria that do not apply to the consideration of the withdrawal of other forms of life support are applied to defend the continuous use of nutrition and hydration; for example, the certainty of death that forbids the withholding of nutrition and hydration is not a factor that forbids the withdrawal of a mechanical ventilator.

Arguments in FAVOR of withholding and withdrawing nutrition and hydration:

Nutrition and hydration are analogous to other life supportive means such as ventilators and should be treated as such, that is, be withheld or withdrawn when the burdens of the treatment outweigh the benefits of the treatment. It is cruel to restrain patients in order to feed them forcibly. Withholding or withdrawing nutrition and hydration is not like killing the patient because if a patient is unable to sit up and eat it is because of the underlying disease (such as a neurological disease). Therefore the patient dies of his own disease when nutrition and hydration are withdrawn; the withdrawal of life support does not kill the patient. Food and fluids may exacerbate distressing symptoms (such as confusion or vomiting) in terminally ill patients; therefore withdrawal of that treatment should remain an option. Debilitated patients could live for 20 years or more on artificial nutrition, which is very expensive care. Symptoms of dehydration and malnutrition after the withdrawal or withholding of nutrition and hydration can be managed through good nursing care (for example, good mouth care).

Implications of choosing this position:

Patients may be more comfortable without artificial tubes and intravenous lines. Patients will retain their ability to choose their treatment as with other forms of life support. Patients with a low quality of life may be seen as expendable. Patients may experience symptoms of dehydration and malnutrition after nutrition and hydration are withdrawn. Money will be saved by not maintaining debilitated patients on artificial nutrition.

Guidelines for the nurse caring for a patient for whom withholding or withdrawal of nutrition and hydration is being considered:

1. Assess the patient for alertness, symptoms of pain and suffering, fluid balance, nutritional state, respirator status and gastrointestinal status. Check the most recent laboratory values. Consult with a dietician and pharmacist, as appropriate.

2. Review the patient's chart and note the reason for admission, history, course of treatment, goals of treatment, advance directives, if any, family situation, DNR order, if any, and reasons why withholding or withdrawal of nutrition and hydration is being considered.

3. Discuss the matter with the patient's physician. Be present at discussions between the patient and the physician as patient advocate.

4. Consider a patient care conference if needed to facilitate communication among those involved in the patient's care and to facilitate an agreement on a plan of care.

5. If a patient care conference does not produce an agreement about the plan of care for the patient, notify your supervisor and consult with the bioethics committee.

6. If nutrition and hydration are to be withheld or withdrawn:

   a. provide emotional support for the patient and family

   b. provide nursing interventions for comfort

   c. ensure that a DNR order is in place

   d. reassess effectiveness of this plan of care and discuss with the physician and patient

   e. If you are uncomfortable with this arrangement, notify your supervisor and find another RN to provide care for the patient.

7. If nutrition and hydration are to be initiated or continued:

   a. provide emotional support for the patient and family

   b. provide nursing interventions for comfort

   c. pay attention to fluid balance, nutrition, GI status

   d. initiate discharge planning, if appropriate

   e. reassess effectiveness of this plan of care and discuss with the physician and patient.

Bibliography

American Nurses' Association. Guidelines on Withdrawing or Withholding Food and Fluid. Ethics in Nursing: Position Statements and Guidelines. Kansas City, Mo.: American Nurses' Association, 1988:2-5.

Barnie DC. Percutaneous Endoscopic Gastrostomy Tubes: The Nurse's role in a Moral, Ethical, and Legal Dilemma. Society of Gastroenterology Nurses and Associates. 1990 Spring:250-254.

Kane FI. Keeping Elizabeth Bouvia Alive for the Public Good. Hastings Center Report,:. 1985 December; 15(6): 5-8.

Lynn J and Childress JF. Must Patients Always be Given Food and Water? Hastings Center Report. 1983, October; 13(5): 17-21

McCormick RA. The *Cruzan* Decision. Midwest Medical Ethics. 1989 Winter/Spring: 6-9.

Meilaender G. The *Cruzan* Decision: A Moral Commentary. Midwest Medical Ethics. 1989 Winter/Spring:6-9.

Meilaender G. On Removing Food and Water: Against the Stream. Hastings Center Report. 1984 December; 14(6): 11-13.

Schmitz P and O'Brien M. Observations on Nutrition and Hydration in Dying Cancer Patients. in By No Extraordinary Means: The Choice to forgo Life-Sustaining Food and Water. Lynn J. (ed). Bloomington, Indiana, Indiana University Press, 1986.

36

Management of Patients with Gastric and Duodenal Disorders

I. Learning Objectives:

In addition to the learning objectives on page 883, I want my students to be able to:

1. _____

2. _____

3. _____

II. Top Terms:

1. Achlorhydria
2. Gastritis
3. H-pylori
4. Morbid Obesity

5. Peptic Ulcer
6. Pyloric Obstruction
7. Pyrosis
8. Zollinger-Ellison Syndrome

III. Collaborative Learning Activities:

Team Discussion Questions/Seminar Topics

1. Discuss the etiology, symptomatology, diagnostic evaluation, medical management and nursing care for patients with Zollinger-Ellison Syndrome.

2. Compare and contrast the differences in duodenal and gastric ulcers according to incidence, symptoms, and risk factors.

IV. Critical Thinking Exercises

In-Class Team Exercise

1. Complete the following chart by listing the major action and nursing consideration for drugs used in duodenal ulcer therapy. (reference pages 889-890, Table 36-2)

Drug Classification	Action	Nursing Considerations
Magnesium Based Antacids		
Cimetidine		
Ranitidine		
Famotidine		
Sucralfate		
Misoprostal		
Pirenzepine		

Send-Home Assignments

Complete the following chart by listing the description and comments for each gastric operation for peptic ulcers. (reference page 892, Table 36-3)

Operation	Description	Comments
Vagotomy		
Truncal Vagotomy		
Selective Vagotomy		
Pyloroplasty		
Billroth I		
Billroth II		

37

Management of Patients with Intestinal and Rectal Disorders

I. Learning Objectives:

In addition to the learning objectives on page 907, I want my students to be able to:

1. _____

2. _____

3. _____

II. Top Terms:

1. Borborymus
2. Crohn's Disease
3. Colonoscopy
4. Diverticulitis
5. Effluent
6. Evisceration
7. Fissure
8. Hirsutism

9. Ileostomy
10. McBurney's Point
11. Megacolon
12. Peritonitis
13. Pilonidal Cyst
14. Polyp
15. Tenesmus
16. Valsalva Maneuver

III. Collaborative Learning Activities:

Team Discussion Questions/Seminar Topics

1. Discuss the physiological processes associated with the act of defecation, including the myoeletric activity.

2. Explain the physiologic processes involved in the Valsalva Maneuver.

3. Locate McBurney's Point on a classmate and explain the concept of "rebound tenderness" as it relates to appendicitis.

IV. Critical Thinking Activities

In-Class Team Exercises

Complete the following crossword puzzle using common terms associated with intestinal and rectal disorders.

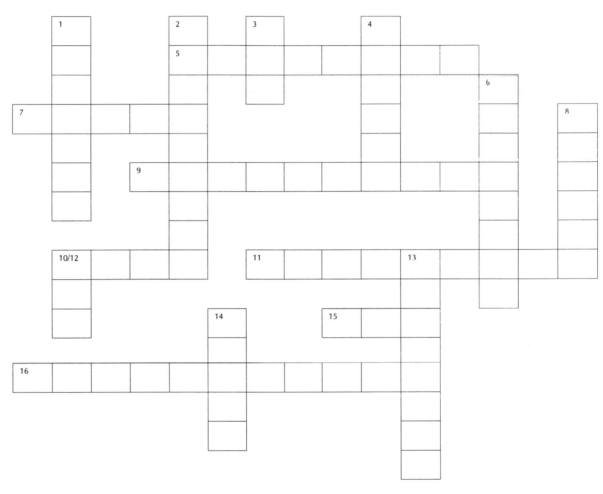

Down

1. A tubular fibrous tract that extends from an opening beside the anus into the anal canal.
2. Dilated and atonic colon caused by a fecal mass.
3. A chemotherapeutic agent used to treat colon cancer.
4. A food to avoid for a patient with an ileostomy.
6. Straining at stool
8. Another name for regional enteritis
12. A highly reliable blood study used to diagnose colon cancer
13. Painful straining at stool
14. The most common bacteria associated with peritonitis.

Across

5. Another term for fecal matter
7. An ileal outlet on the abdomen
9. Intestinal rumbling
10. Another food to avoid for a patient with an ileostomy
11. The most popular "over-the-counter" medications purchased in the U.S.
15. Intravenous nutrition used for inflammatory bowel disease
16. The most common complication of appendicitis.

Send-Home Assignments

Complete the following chart for each of the six classifications of laxatives. (reference page 909, Table 37-1)

Classification	Prototype	Action	Potential Side-Effects	Patient Education
Bulk-Forming				
Saline				
Lubricant				
Stimulant				
Fecal Softener				
Osmotic Agent				

ETHICAL QUESTION: SHOULD PATIENTS WITH "SELF-INFLICTED" LIVER DISEASE RECEIVE LIVER TRANSPLANTS?

Discussion: Liver disease can develop secondary to drug and alcohol abuse. Should patients with this so-called "self-inflicted" disease be considered along with "innocent" victims of liver disease for rare liver transplants? Should patients with idiopathic liver disease receive preference for organs over patients with self-inflicted disease?

Dilemma: The patient's desire for treatment of his disease conflicts with obligation to distribute scarce resources in a fair manner (autonomy versus justice).

Arguments that patients with self-inflicted liver disease SHOULD be considered for liver transplants: Substance abuse is a disease; therefore, liver disease secondary to drug or alcohol abuse is not self-inflicted and these patients should be considered along with all other eligible patients for organ transplants. Health care professionals are not qualified to judge the worthiness of patients for transplantation and therefore should not be in the position of doing so. Excluding patients from life-saving organ transplants simply because of a history of drug or alcohol abuse constitutes a prejudice and is not just.

Implications of choosing this position: Some transplanted livers may be given to patients who return to substance abuse behavior and do not cooperate with the post-transplant regimen. Patients with "innocent" liver disease may be passed over for organ transplant.

Arguments that patients with self-inflicted liver disease SHOULD NOT be considered for liver transplants: It is not just to give scarce organs to patients who will abuse and damage the transplanted organ. Substance abuse behavior should not be rewarded. Substance abuse patients will not cooperate with the post-transplant regimen. The scarcity of organs demands strict criteria for transplant recipients and therefore it is just to exclude those with self-inflicted disease.

Implications of choosing this position: Patients who would otherwise qualify for liver transplants would be excluded because of history of substance abuse. Some patients with "innocent" liver disease may not follow the post-transplant regimen.

Potential Compromise: Consider all patients with liver disease from all causes for liver transplants, but use as one exclusionary criterion the best judgment about a patient's ability to follow through with the post-operative treatment regimen. Those patients who are judged as unlikely to follow the postoperative regimen should not be considered for a liver transplant.

Implications of choosing this position: Estimate of which patients will be able to follow the post-operative regimen is only a guess and that guess may be based on prejudice about substance abuse history.

Guidelines for the nurse caring for a patient with end-stage alcoholic liver cirrhosis who may be a possible candidate for liver transplant:

1. Review the chart for the patient's history, course of treatment, and current state of disease. Was the patient abusing alcohol or drugs recently? Does he attend AA or other therapy or recovery process?

2. Assess the patient's knowledge level about liver disease, the liver transplant procedure and the post-operative regimen. Document this information in the chart.

3. Assess, monitor and document the patient's ability and interest in following the medical regimen.

4. Discuss the patient's case with the physician. Discover if the patient is being considered for a liver transplant, and if not, why not.

5. Research the hospital's or local transplant consortium's policy on liver transplants for substance abusers. Is the policy a good and fair one?

6. If the physician's rationale for denying the patient for consideration for a liver transplant conflicts with the policy, discuss this with him. Suggest a patient care conference or a bioethics committee consultation to discuss the issue further.

Bibliography

O'Connell DA. Ethical Implications of Organ Transplantation. Critical Care Nurse Quarterly. 1991 February; 13(4): 1-7.

Olbrish ME and Levenson JL. Liver Transplantation for Alcoholic Cirrhosis. Journal of the American Medical Association. 1989 May 26; 261(20): 2958.

Omery A and Caswell D. A Nursing Perspective of the Ethical Issues Surrounding Liver Transplantation. Heart and Lung. 1988 November; 17(6): 626-681.

Starzl TE. et. al. Orthotopic Liver Transplantation for Alcoholic Cirrhosis. Journal of the American Medical Association. 1988 November 4; 260(17): 2542-2544.

Sheets L. Liver Transplantation. Nurs Clin North Am. 1989 December, 24(4). 881-889.

Instructional Improvement Tool for Unit

Student feedback/evaluation indicated that I need to improve my classroom presentation by:

Adding Content

1. _____
   _____
2. _____
   _____
3. _____
   _____

Deleting Content

1. _____
   _____
2. _____
   _____
3. _____
   _____

Emphasizing/De-emphasizing the Following Content

1. _____
   _____
2. _____
   _____
3. _____
   _____

Questions students asked that I need to research for the future are:

1. _____
   _____
   _____
2. _____
   _____
3. _____
   _____

38

Assessment and Management of Patients with Hepatic and Biliary Disorders

I. Learning Objectives:

In addition to the learning objectives on page 959, I want my students to be able to:

1. _____

2. _____

3. _____

II. Top Terms:

1. Ascites
2. Asterixis
3. Canaliculi
4. Caput Medusae
5. Cholecystectomy
6. Encephalopathy
7. Fetor Hepaticas

8. Gluconeogenesis
9. Glycogen
10. Hepatocytes
11. Lithotripsy
12. Portacaval Anastomosis
13. Spider Telangiectasis
14. Urobilinogen

III. Collaborative Learning Activities:

Team Discussion Questions/Seminar Topics

1. Select a group of students to present the pathophysiologic processes that result in the body retaining increased amounts of ammonia which lead to hepatic coma.

2. Assign several students to explain the process of extracorporeal shock-wave lithotripsy, including a patient teaching plan for pre-treatment preparation.

3. Encourage a discussion of the factors that put individuals "at-risk" for Hepatitis B and suggest that a team of students present a list of preventive measures.

IV. Critical Thinking Exercises

In-Class Team Exercises

1. List in numerical order the sequence of events leading from portal hypertension to ascites formation and generalized fluid retention. (reference pages 971-972 [Figure 38-5])

   a. Ascites

   b. Decreased intravascular fluid volume

   c. Increased aldosterone secretion by the adrenal glands

   d. Retention of sodium and water by kidneys to increase intravascular fluid volume

   e. Obstruction to the flow of portal venous blood through the liver

   f. Portal hypertension throughout entire portal venous system

   g. Release of renin by the kidneys

   (1) _____   (5) _____

   (2) _____   (6) _____

   (3) _____   (7) _____

   (4) _____

2. Next to each of the abnormal liver function studies (normal values found on textbook pages 965-967), list a possible rationale for each reading and any associated clinical manifestations. (reference page 964 [Table 38-1])

Abnormal Study	Rationale	Clinical Manifestations
Total serum bilirubin of 1.8 mg/dl.		
Alkaline phosphatase of 6.5 u/dl (Bodansky method)		
A blood ammonia level of 100 mg/dl		
Total serum protein of 5.5 gm/dl		
Serum glutamic-oxaloacetic transaminase (SGOT) of 60 units		
Serum glutamic-pyruvic transaminase (SGPT) of 60 units		

Send-Home Assignments

Complete the following chart comparing the five types of Hepatitis including implications for patient education. (reference pages 976-983, Table 38-3)

	Hepatitis A	Hepatitis B	Hepatitis C	Hepatitis D	Hepatitis E
Etiology					
Transmission					
Incubation					
Immunity					
Patient Teaching Guidelines					

Compare and contrast the following three types of jaundice with respect to etiology, pathophysiology, and clinical manifestations. (reference pages 970-971)

Jaundice	Etiology	Pathophysiology	Clinical Manifestations
Hemolytic			
Hepatocellular			
Obstructive			

39

Assessment and Management
of Patients with Diabetes Mellitus

I. Learning Objectives:

In addition to the learning objectives on page 1015, I want my students to be able to:

1. _____

2. _____

3. _____

II. Top Terms:

1. Flocculation
2. Gestational Diabetes
3. Glycemia Index
4. Hypoglycemia
5. Islet Cells
6. Ketoacidosis
7. Ketonuria
8. Kussmaul Respirations
9. Lipodystrophy
10. Lipohypertrophy
11. Paresthesia
12. Polyuria
13. Retinopathy
14. SMGB
15. Somogyi Effect
16. Vitrectomy

III. Collaborative Learning Activities:

Team Discussion Questions/Seminar Topics

1. Present an outline of the epidemiology of Diabetes Mellitus, the third leading cause of death in the U.S.

2. Describe the clinical concerns of a patient who is pregnant and has diabetes.

3. Explain why exercise is not recommended for patients with diabetes whose blood glucose level is over 250 mg/dl (14 mmol/L) and who have ketonuria.

4. Describe the clinical picture of someone with hyperosmolar, nonketotoxic syndrome (HNKS).

5. Draft an outline of the current treatment protocol for diabetic retinopathy.

IV. Critical Thinking Activities

In-Class Team Exercises

1. Assign a group of students the development of a patient teaching guide for a 50-year-old woman to self-administer insulin subcutaneously. In the space provided, develop a teaching plan that will meet the following goals and actions. (reference pages 1033-1037 [Chart 39-3 and 39-4])

   a. Withdrawal of 20 units of NPH insulin from a vial

   b. Preparation of the skin

   c. Insertion of the needle, aspiration, and injection

   d. Rotation of sites

   e. Care of the equipment

2. Develop preoperative and postoperative nursing management checklists for a diabetic patient who is to undergo surgery. These would supplement the routine checklists used in clinical settings. For each area to be assessed, cite the rationale for assessment and list the expected physiological alteration. (reference pages 1058-1061)

Preoperative Nursing Management

Area	Rationale	Expected Physiological Alteration

Postoperative Nursing Management

Area	Rationale	Expected Physiological Alteration

Send-Home Assignments

1. Compare and contrast the two most common types of diabetes according to etiology, pathophysiology and clinical manifestations. (reference pages 1016-1020 and Table 39-1)

Type	Etiology	Pathophysiology	Clinical Manifestations
Type I: Insulin-dependent diabetes mellitus			
Type II: Non-insulin dependent diabetes mellitus			

2. Construct a nursing care plan for a 30-year-old person with diabetes who has been insulin dependent for 16 years and needs 27 units of lente insulin daily. She is moderately active, is restricted to a 2000-calorie American Diabetic Association diet, and smokes one pack of cigarettes per day. She lives at home with her husband and two children. She is beginning to show signs of retinopathy. (reference pages 1028-1036)

Nursing Diagnosis:

Immediate Goal:

Intermediate Goal:

Long-Term Goal:

Nursing Intervention   **Expected Outcomes**

3. Paula, a 36-year-old woman with diabetes, is using an insulin pump system (continuous subcutaneous insulin infusion). She works at home in her husband's dental office and is the mother of 8-year-old twin girls. (reference pages 59-61)

a. Compare the advantages and disadvantages of an insulin pump system.

Advantages: **Disadvantages:**

b. Develop a teaching plan for Paula to teach her how to use an insulin pump. Use the following format:

Specific Teaching Points   **Rationale**

40

Assessment and Management of Patients with Endocrine Disorders

I. Learning Objectives:

In addition to the learning objectives on page 1069, I want my students to be able to:

1. _____

2. _____

3. _____

II. Top Terms:

1. Basal Metabolic Rate
2. Diabetes Insipidus
3. Exocrine Gland
4. Feedback Control
5. Exophthalmos

6. Feedback Control
7. Goiter
8. Grave's Disease
9. Hormone
10. Whipple Procedure

III. Collaborative Learning Activities:

Team Discussion Questions/Seminar Topics

1. Explain the differences in structure and function of the endocrine and exocrine glands.

2. Support the following statement with a rationale explanation. "The pituitary gland is the *master gland* of the endocrine system."

3. Explain why there is an increased incidence of angina pectoris or myocardial infarction as a response to therapy for myxedema.

IV. Critical Thinking Activities

In-Class Team Exercises

1. Compare and contrast the etiology, clinical manifestations, medical management and nursing interventions for diabetes insipidus and diabetes mellitus. (reference pages 1104-1105 and Chapter 39)

	Etiology	Clinical Manifestations	Medical Management	Nursing Intervention
Diabetes Insipidus				
Diabetes Mellitus				

2. Outline the concept of the negative feedback mechanism for hypothalmic-pituitary interactions as illustrated below in Figure 40-4.

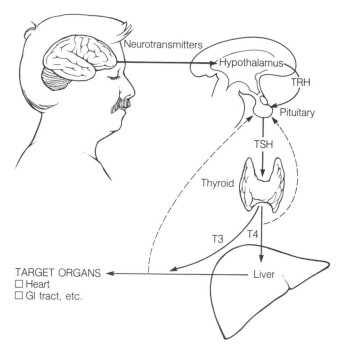

Figure 40-4. The hypothalmic-pituitary-thyroid axis.

Send-Home Assignments

Read the following case study. Fill in the blanks or circle the correct answer.

Case Study: Hyperparathyroidism

Emily is a 65-year-old who has been complaining of continued emotional irritability. Her family described her as always "on edge" and neurotic. After several months of exacerbated symptoms, Emily underwent a complete physical examination and was diagnosed with hyperparathyroidism. (reference pages 1091-1092)

1. Emily's clinical symptoms are all related to an increase in serum:

   a. calcium.

   b. magnesium.

   c. potassium.

   d. sodium.

2. As a nurse you know that the normal levels of the mineral identified above are:

   a. 8.8 to 10 mg/dl.

   b. 1.3 to 2.1 mEq /L

   c. 3.5 to 5 mEq/L

   d. 135 to 148 mmol/L

3. Describe eight symptoms usually seen when hyperparathyroidism involves several body systems:

   a. _____   e. _____

   b. _____   f. _____

   c. _____   g. _____

   d. _____   h. _____

4. Name one of the most important organ complications of hyperparathyroidism.

5. A musculoskeletal symptom(s) found with hyperparathyroidism is:

   a. deformities due to demineralization.

   b. pain on weight-bearing.

   c. pathologic fractures due to osteoclast growth.

   d. all of the above may occur.

6. The recommended treatment for primary hyperparathyroidism is:

   a. pharmacotherapy until the elevated serum levels return to normal.

   b. surgical removal of the abnormal parathyroid tissue.

   c. adrenalectomy.

   d. all of the above treatments are recommended.

7. Acute hypercalcemic crises can occur in hyperparathyroidism. The treatment would involve immediate:

   a. administration of diuretic agents to promote renal excretion of calcium.

   b. phosphate therapy to correct hypophosphatemia.

   c. rehydration with large volumes of intravenous fluids.

   d. management with all of the above modalities.

Instructional Improvement Tool for Unit

Student feedback/evaluation indicated that I need to improve my classroom presentation by:

Adding Content

1. _____

_____

2. _____

_____

3. _____

_____

Deleting Content

1. _____

_____

2. _____

_____

3. _____

_____

Emphasizing/De-emphasizing the Following Content

1. _____

_____

2. _____

_____

3. _____

_____

Questions students asked that I need to research for the future are:

1. _____

_____

_____

2. _____

_____

3. _____

_____

41

Assessment of Urinary and Renal Function

I. Learning Objectives:

In addition to the learning objectives on page 1125, I want my students to be able to:

1. _____

2. _____

3. _____

II. Top Terms:

1. Azotemia
2. Enuresis
3. Nephron
4. Nocturia

5. Oliguria
6. Osmolality
7. Urea
8. Uremia

III. Collaborative Learning Activities:

Team Discussion Questions/Seminar Topics

1. Outline the nursing actions needed to prepare a patient for a cystoscopic examination.

2. Compare and contrast the purpose and patient preparation needed for those undergoing an ultrasound, a KUB x-ray and an MRI for kidney function assessment.

IV. Critical Thinking Activities

In-Class Team Exercises

For each term that describes a voiding problem, list a potential cause and associated nursing assessment activities. (reference page 1134, Chart 41-1)

Voiding Concern	Potential Cause	Nursing Assessment
Dysuria		
Nocturia		
Hesitancy		
Stress Incontinence		
Proteinuria		
Polyuria		

Send-Home Assignments

Develop a nursing care plan for a patient who is scheduled for a renal biopsy. Include post-biopsy nursing management guidelines. (reference pages 1137-1138)

42

Management of Patients with Urinary and Renal Dysfunction

I. Learning Objectives:

In addition to the learning objectives on page 1145, I want my students to be able to:

1. _____

2. _____

3. _____

II. Top Terms:

1. Atony
2. CAPD
3. Dialysis
4. Dialysate
5. Fistula
6. Hemofiltration

7. Peritoneal Dialysis
8. Residual Urine
9. Shunt
10. Stress Incontinence
11. Trocar
12. Ureteral Stent

III. Collaborative Learning Activities:

Team Discussion Questions/Seminar Topics

1. Discuss nursing measures to prevent microorganisms from gaining access to the urinary tract by each of the three most common routes.

2. Describe the procedure and patient preparation needed for a patient with suprapubic bladder drainage.

3. Discuss the rationale behind a liberal fluid intake with catheterization as a nursing measure for treatment of neurogenic bladder.

4. Explain the concept and process of "high-flux" dialysis.

IV. Critical Thinking Activities

In-Class Team Exercises

1. Describe 10 out of 18 ways nurses can prevent and control infection in catheterized patients. (reference pages 1149, Chart 42-2)

2. For each of the four causes of urinary incontinence, outline management interventions and nursing care activities. (reference pages 1151-1152)

Type of Urinary Incontinence	Medical Management Strategies	Nursing Interventions
Stress Incontinence		
Urge Incontinence		
Overflow Incontinence		
Functional Incontinence		

Send-Home Assignments

Examine Figure 42-4. Describe the process of dialysis as illustrated in the figure, making sure to mention the principles underlying the process. Develop a nursing care plan that addresses patient teaching guidelines for management of a patient on long-term hemodialysis. (reference page 1156)

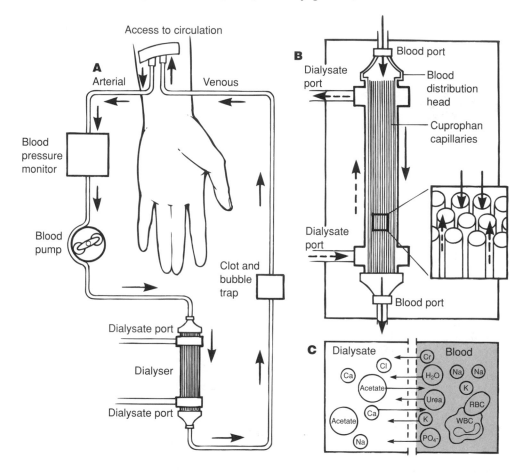

Figure 42-4

ETHICAL QUESTION. SHOULD THERE BE LIMITS ON THE USE OF DIALYSIS?

Discussion: Hemodialysis is an expensive but life-saving procedure that is currently being used for more than 100,000 Americans. For some, hemodialysis allows them to live near-normal lives despite the kidney failure that would otherwise kill them. Other patients have a less optimistic outlook. Some patients with multiple system organ failure are given hemodialysis that serves to merely prolong their dying process. Since dialysis is an expensive procedure in an age when costs are being scrutinized carefully, it is reasonable to ask if dialysis should be rationed. Some ways in which dialysis can be rationed are by age, by HIV status, by quality of life, or by ability to pay.

Dilemma: The demand of the patient for life-saving treatment conflicts with the public's need to provide and pay for the most cost-effective treatment for all (autonomy versus justice).

Arguments that there SHOULD be limits on dialysis: Dialysis is expensive, and significant savings will result from rationing it. A fair means for rationing can be found, for example: no dialysis for people over 80; no dialysis for HIV positive patients. As long as standards are adhered to, everyone will be treated the same. Health care providers have shown themselves to be prone to rationing unfairly (see bibliography), therefore standards need to be imposed.

Implications of choosing this position: Savings will result from rationing dialysis. Patients will die without dialysis, some of whom could have lived fruitful lives with dialysis. There will be a public outcry over any rationing standard and negative publicity regarding those denied dialysis. There is a risk of engaging the slippery slope, for example, reducing the age at which dialysis can be started and then not giving dialysis to someone with a perceived poor quality of life.

Arguments that there SHOULD NOT be limits on dialysis: There are no limits on other life-support systems. Therefore, why should there be limits for dialysis? All standards for rationing dialysis will eventually deteriorate into subjective quality of life standards, that is, the standards cannot be made fair or stay fair. Patient conditions and circumstances vary considerably; it is difficult to use one criterion for excluding patients (that is, some elderly patients could benefit from dialysis, as could some HIV positive patients).

Implications of choosing this position: Without limits, money will continue to be spent on dialysis treatments that may or may not benefit patients. Money spent on dialyzing patients who do not benefit from it will not be available for more cost-effective care, such as pre-natal care. To choose this position is to admit that any type of rationing will be ineffective or unfair.

Potential compromise: Have professional organizations agree to objective standards for dialysis, such as an age limit, or an age limit combined with an assessment of the patient's overall degree of health or illness. Avoid attempts to quantify quality of life, though considerations of the patient's compliance with treatment may be appropriate. Government organizations should earmark monetary savings for another program such as pre-natal care.

Implications of choosing this position: Professionally-developed standards may be adhered to more successfully than governmental standards. The problems with rationing — deaths, public outcry — are still involved, as are problems with maintaining standards.

Bibliography

Bayer R. et. al. The Care of the Terminally Ill: Morality and Economics. New England Journal of Medicine. 1983 December 15; 309(24):1490-1494.

Bermel J. The Pheonix Memo: Rationing Dialysis for [American] Indian Patients. Hastings Center Report. 1983 April; 13(2): 2.

Callahan D. Allocating Health Resources. Hastings Center Report. 1988 April-May; 18(2): 14- 20.

Callahan D. Setting Limits: Medical Goals in an Aging Society. N.Y., Touchstone/Simon and Schuster, 1987.

Johnson DE. Life, Death and the Dollar Sign: Medical Ethics and Cost Containment. Journal of the American Medical Association. 1984 July 13; 252(2): 223-224.

Levine C. Stopping Dialysis for 'Low Quality of Life' : A Case from Britain. Hastings Center Report. 1985 February; 15(l): 2-3.

Neu S. and Kjellstrand CM. Stopping Long Term Dialysis: An Empirical Study of Withdrawal of Life-Saving Treatment. New England Journal of Medicine. 1986 January 2; 314(l): 14-16.

Scott J. Ethical Issues: A Washington Perspective. Nursing Management. 1992 January; 23(l):52-56.

43

Management of Patients with Urinary and Renal Disorders

I. Learning Objectives:

In addition to the learning objectives on page 1179, I want my students to be able to:

1. _____

2. _____

3. _____

II. Top Terms:

1. Bacteria
2. Cystitis
3. Cystotomy
4. Interstitial Cystitis
5. Lithotripsy

6. Nephrectomy
7. Nephrosclerosis
8. Ureterostomy
9. Urethrovesical Reflex
10. UTI

III. Collaborative Learning Activities:

Team Discussion Questions/Seminar Topics

1. Draft an outline of a patient teaching guide to help a patient decrease the incidence of recurring urinary tract infections.

2. Compare and contrast the differences between chronic and acute glomerulonephritis relative to etiology, clinical manifestations, diagnostic evaluation, medical management, and nursing interventions.

IV. Critical Thinking Activities

In-Class Team Exercises

Consider a patient who has been diagnosed with renal stones. The physician has prescribed *Extracorporeal Shock Wave Lithotripsy*. Use the following three nursing diagnoses and develop a nursing care plan for a 46-year-old oil company executive who needs treatment away from home. (reference pages 1211-1213)

Nursing Diagnoses: Pain related to inflammation, obstruction, and abrasion of the urinary tract.

Knowledge deficit regarding prevention of recurrence of renal stones.

Risk for loneliness related to separation from family.

Potential Complications: Infection and sepsis

Obstruction of the urinary tract by a stone or edema with subsequent acute renal failure.

Send-Home Assignments

Examine Figure 43-7 (A) and complete the following case study. Circle the correct answer. (Reference pages 1217-1220)

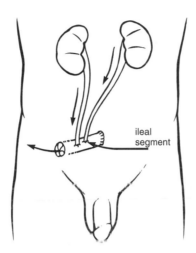

Figure 43-7(A) Ileal conduit ureters transplanted to section of ileum and brought out opening in abdominal wall

Read the following case study. Circle the correct answer.

Case Study: Ileal Conduit

Gregory, a 69-year-old widower, has just undergone an ileal conduit. He came back to the clinical area 24 hours postoperatively.

1. In preparation for postoperative management, the nurse understands that an ileal conduit involves:

    a. bringing a detached ureter through the abdominal wall and through a skin opening.

    b. inserting a catheter into the renal pelvis through an incision into the flank.

    c. introducing the ureter into the sigmoid, thus allowing urine to flow through the colon and onto the abdomen.

    d. transplanting the ureters to an isolated section of the terminal ileum and bringing one end to the abdominal wall.

2. After initial postoperative assessment, the nurse should do all of the following *except*:

   a. check the skin around the stoma for encrustation with dermatitis.

   b. encourage a soft, high-fiber diet for the first 3 postoperative days.

   c. inspect the stoma for bleeding.

   d. measure hourly urinary outputs.

3. The nurse frequently assesses the stomal mucosa for peristomal dermatitis, which can be avoided by maintaining a urine pH:

   a. below 6.5.

   b. around 7.0.

   c. between 7.0 and 7.5.

   d. above 8.0.

4. The nurse needs to teach Gregory to empty the ostomy appliance:

   a. before sleep so that urine does not flow backward into the abdomen.

   b. every 2 hours in an effort to control odor by frequently draining the system.

   c. twice a day, to minimize infection by decreasing the frequency of opening the valve.

   d. when it is about half full, to prevent separation of the unit from the stoma because of the increased weight caused by the urine.

5. The ostomy appliance needs to be changed every 5 to 7 days. Gregory needs to know that he should:

   a. bend over and empty the conduit before the skin is washed and dried.

   b. pat the skin dry so that the appliance will adhere.

   c. center the appliance over the stoma and apply gentle pressure to remove air bubbles and creases.

   d. do all of the above.

Instructional Improvement Tool for Unit

Student feedback/evaluation indicated that I need to improve my classroom presentation by:

Adding Content

1. _____
   _____

2. _____
   _____

3. _____
   _____

Deleting Content

1. _____
   _____

2. _____
   _____

3. _____
   _____

Emphasizing/De-emphasizing the Following Content

1. _____
   _____

2. _____
   _____

3. _____
   _____

Questions students asked that I need to research for the future are:

1. _____
   _____
   _____

2. _____
   _____

3. _____
   _____

44

Assessment and Management of Patients with Problems Related to Female Physiologic Processes

I. Learning Objectives:

In addition to the learning objectives on page 1233, I want my students to be able to:

1. _____

2. _____

3. _____

II. Top Terms:

1. Bartholin's Gland
2. Chadwick's Sign
3. Coloscopy
4. Cystocele
5. Douches
6. Endometrium

7. Hysteroscopy
8. Insufflation
9. Laparoscopy
10. Menopause
11. Menstruation
12. Ovulation

III. Collaborative Learning Activities:

Team Discussion Questions/Seminar Topics

1. Compare and contrast the signs and symptoms of primary and secondary dysmenorrhea. Offer several suggestions for management of symptoms.

2. Compare and contrast two sterilization methods, vasectomy and laparoscopic tubal sterilization. Outline ethical issues that might be discussed by patients prior to making these decisions. What is the scope of the nurse's role in advising?

IV. Critical Thinking Exercises

In-Class Team Exercises

Mark 28 days on a linear graph. List the five phases of endometrial changes (menstrual, follicular, ovulation, luteal, and premenstrual) over the approximate number of days. For each cycle, distinguish between the expected changes in the ovary and the endometrium, and the secretion levels of estrogen, FSH and LH. (reference page 1247 and Table 44-2)

Phase _____

Days _____

Changes: _____

Send-Home Assignments

Diagnostic Diary

Keep a personal three month menstrual cycle diary (or give the diary to someone to complete) using the form below (Figure 44-8). When the data is complete, examine the data to determine if there is any repetitive pattern. If so, then develop a teaching guide with recommendations for managing the symptoms relative to diet and exercise. (reference pages 1247-1248)

Diagnostic Diary A: Evaluation of PMS Symptoms

NAME _____

YEAR _____

Grading of Symptoms:
0—*No Symptoms*   2—*Moderate Symptoms*
1—*Mild Symptoms*   3—*Severe Symptoms (i.e., Disabling)*

DAY OF CYCLE	1	2	3	4	5	6	7	8	9	10	11	12	13	14	15	16	17	18	19	20	21	22	23	24	25	26	27	28	29	30	31
DATE																															
MENSES																															

PSYCHOLOGICAL SYMPTOMS

Depression																															
Anxiety																															
Irritability																															
Lethargy																															
Insomnia																															
Forgetfulness																															
Confusion																															

PHYSICAL SYMPTOMS

Swelling																															
Breast Tenderness																															
Abdominal bloating																															
Palpitations																															
Weight gain																															
Constipation																															
Headache																															
Rhinitis																															

PAIN SYMPTOMS (Usually NOT associated with PMS)

Menstrual cramps																															
Painful intercourse																															
Pelvic pain																															
Backache																															

Morning weight (lb)																															

Figure 44-8. Diagnostic diary for evaluation of PMS symptoms. (Chihal HJ. Premenstrual Syndrome: A Clinic Manual, 2nd ed. Dallas, Essential Medical Information Systems, 1990, pp 80-81.)

ETHICAL QUESTION: SHOULD ABORTION BE LEGAL?

Discussion: At conception, a genetically unique human blueprint is formed. Allowing for the 25% of all pregnancies which will end in miscarriage, 75% of all fertilized eggs will, if allowed to grow, result in the birth of a human baby. Should the mother have the right to medical services which would allow her to terminate her pregnancy? The debate over whether the fetus is a human being and whether women should have a legal right to choose an abortion has raged for over 30 years and has dominated American laws, politics and headlines. The debate has become so personal and fractious that it has become difficult for opposite sides to have a civilized discussion about the issue. Often the two sides cannot agree on the terminology to use in the debate. In a good ethical debate, the terminology should be neutral and the pros and cons of each position should be examined.

Dilemma: The freedom of a competent adult woman to choose whether or not to undergo an abortion conflicts with the life, growth, and development of the genetically unique human within her. The debate could be described as the mother's versus the baby's interests., or autonomy versus beneficence. The debate could also be characterized as the baby's interests in life conflicting with what is just and right for women in general, or autonomy versus justice. A third way of describing the debate is the mother's interests versus the baby's interests, or autonomy versus autonomy. Different factions characterize the debate in different ways.

Arguments FOR abortion being legal: Women would be treated as less than competent, adult citizens if they did not have the right to choose to terminate their pregnancy. The desire to terminate a pregnancy for some women is so strong that these women will resort to illegal abortions if legal abortions are not available; thus making abortions illegal will result in the death of women from illegal, unsterile and unsafe abortions. The moral position of the fetus should not be held as highly as that of the mother because: the fetus is not yet human because it is not yet fully developed, the fetus cannot survive outside the mother's womb, and the mother is a competent adult. Society does not provide support for pregnant women and women with children, therefore it is a great financial burden on women to be forced to go through with a pregnancy. A woman should not be forced to carry an unwanted or deformed fetus to term.

Implications of choosing this position: Legal abortion services make it possible for abortions to be performed for morally disreputable reasons such as sex selection or birth control. Acceptance of legal abortions may contribute to the view that some life is expendable. There will be fewer children available for adoption. Abortions would be relatively safe, clean and sterile. A few women would die from abortions despite legal services. The availability of abortion services might encourage some women to abort who might otherwise have carried their babies to term.

Argument AGAINST legalized abortion: The fetus is alive and is therefore a human life that should be respected and protected. Neither women nor men should have the right to terminate human life for reasons of convenience, sex selection or birth control reasons. Handicapped children are human beings and deserve to live. The unavailability of abortions will encourage women to carry their babies to term.

Implications of choosing this position: The numbers of abortions will be reduced. The numbers of births of normal and abnormal children will increase. There will be more children available for adoption. There will be more unwanted children. There will be an increased financial burden on women with children. Some women will resort to illegal and unsafe abortions and some women will die from their use of these services. A black market in abortion services may arise. Women with financial resources, but not poor women, may be able to gain access to safe but illegal abortions.

Potential compromise: Restricted abortions. Restrict abortion access to women in their first trimester only, for example.

Implications of choosing this position:	Does not satisfy the objections of either side: fetuses will still die; some women would be denied access to safe and legal abortions. It would satisfy some requirements of each side though by maintaining safe, legal abortion services and reducing the number of abortions.

Guidelines for the nurse caring for a woman undergoing an elective abortion:

1. If you have a moral objection to abortions, you should notify your supervisor and find another nurse to care for the patient.

2. Satisfy yourself that the patient has given informed consent for the abortion and that the abortion coincides with the policies and procedures of your institution and the laws of your state. If not, notify the physician and your supervisor.

3. Provide emotional support for the patient. Avoid judgmental or political comments. Avoid trite comments or platitudes.

Bibliography

Davis SE. Pro-Choice: A New Militancy. Hastings Center Report. 1989 November-December; 19(6): 32-33.

Glendon MA. A World without Roe: How Different Would it Be? Hastings Center Report. 1989 July-August; 19(4): 30-37.

Kaufman F. The Fetus's Mother. Hastings Center Report. 1990 May-June; 20(3): 3-4.

Kennedy BJ. I'm Sorry, Baby. Am J Nurs. 1988 August; 88(8): 1067-1069.

Mahowald ME. Is There Life after Roe v. Wade? Hastings Center Report. 1989 July-August; 19(4): 22-29.

Nathanson B. Operation Rescue: Terrorism or Legitimate Civil Rights Protest? Hastings Center Report. 1989 November-December; 19(6): 28-32.

Thomasma DC. Human Life in the Balance. Louisville, Kentucky, Westminster/John Knox Press, 1990.

ETHICAL QUESTION: SHOULD UNIMPLANTED EMBRYOS BE DISCARDED?

Discussion: Hyperstimulation of the ovaries normally precedes in-vitro fertilization (IVF) in order to obtain an optimum number of eggs. These eggs are then mixed with sperm to produce fertilized eggs for implantation into the infertile female. However, in order to avoid a multiple pregnancy, only a certain number of embryos are implanted at any one time; the rest are frozen. If the implanted embryos grow and result in a successful pregnancy, the remaining embryos may never be used by the woman. What should be done with the remaining embryos? Should they remain frozen forever? Be discarded? Be donated to another infertile couple? Be used for research? What is the status of those embryos?

Dilemma: The obligation to respect and preserve human life conflicts with the mother's right to control her family size and the destiny of her genetic material (beneficence versus autonomy).

Arguments in FAVOR of discarding unused embryos: The embryos are not human life, just potential human life. There is only a very small likelihood that the embryo, even if implanted, would result in a live birth. The parents should have the right to decide about their own family size and the fate of their own genetic material.

Implications of choosing this position: If discarding embryos were not an option, all embryos would have to be implanted in the mother, which would put her at risk of a multiple pregnancy which may be risky for her and for the babies. Or, if discarding embryos were not an option, unimplanted embryos would either have to be frozen forever or donated to another couple or used for experimentation, options that may not be palatable to the parents. Embryos will be seen as expendable.

Arguments AGAINST discarding unused embryos: Embryos are equivalent to human life and should be treated as such. Embryos should be respected and protected, not discarded when their existence is of no use. When parents commit to an IVF treatment, they commit to caring for all the human life that may result. Unimplanted embryos should be kept frozen or donated to another couple.

Implications of choosing this position: Parents using IVF treatments would be committing potentially to a large family, when that may not be what they want at all. The problem of what to do with unused embryos still exists. A perpetually frozen existence does not seem to be a better option than discarding the embryos. Many parents may not want to donate their genetic embryos to another couple. Embryos left in limbo have resulted in custody or other legal battles.

Guidelines for the nurse caring for a couple considering IVF:

1. Assess the couple's knowledge level about IVF and initiate teaching about the procedure and its implications.

2. Encourage the physician and the couple to plan ahead for what to do with unused embryos and document this in the chart.

Bibliography

Annas GJ. Redefining Parenthood and Protecting Embryos: Why we Need New Laws. Hastings Center Report. 1984 October; 14(5):50-52.

The Ethics Committee of the American Fertility Society. Ethical Considerations of the New Reproductive Technologies: the Moral and Legal Status of the Preembryo. Fertility and Sterility. 1990 June Special Supplement; 53(6): 34S-36S.

Grobstein C. The Moral Uses of 'Spare' Embryos. Hastings Center Report. 1982 June; 12(3): 5- 6.

McCormick RA. Who or What is the Pre-Embryo? Kennedy Institute of Ethics Journal. 1991 March; l(l): 1-15.

McCormick RA. The Pre-Embryo as Potential: A Reply to John A. Robertson. Kennedy Institute of Ethics Journal. 1991 December; 1(4): 303-305.

Ozar DT. The Case Against Thawing Unused Frozen Embryos. Hastings Center Report. 1935 August; 5(4): 7-12.

Robertson JA. Resolving Disputes over Frozen Embryos. Hastings Center Report. 1989 November-December; 19(6): 7-12.

Roberston JA. What We May Do with Pre-Embryos: A Response to Richard A. McCormick. Kennedy Institute of Ethics Journal. 1991 December; 1(4): 293-302.

45

Management of Patients with Disorders of the Female Reproductive System

I. Learning Objectives:

In addition to the learning objectives on page 1269, I want my students to be able to:

1. _____

2. _____

3. _____

II. Top Terms:

1. Bartholin's Cyst
2. Candidiasis
3. Cytology
4. Doderlein's Bacillus
5. Dyspareunia
6. Endometriosis
7. Fibroid
8. Genital Herpes
9. Hysterectomy
10. Kegal Exercises
11. Leukorrhea
12. Pessary
13. PID
14. Pruritus
15. Toxic Shock Syndrome
16. Vaginitis
17. Vulvectomy
18. Vulvovaginal Infection

III. Collaborative Learning Activities:

Team Discussion Questions/Seminar Topics

1. Explain why stress increases a women's chance of having a vaginal infection.

2. Describe at least six risk factors for vulvovaginal infections and list two preventive measures for each factor.

3. Compare and contrast the etiology and clinical manifestations of a cystolcele versus a rectocele.

4. Explain what Kegel exercises are and why they are important.

5. Describe the risk factors associated with cancer of the uterus.

IV. Critical Thinking Activities:

In-Class Team Exercises

Read the following case studies. Fill in the blanks or circle the correct answer.

Case Study: Pelvic Inflammatory Disease (PID)

Donna is a 26-year-old graduate student who has been sexually active with multiple partners for five years. Last year she experienced several incidences of cervicitis. She now believes she has PID. (reference pages 1278-1280 and Chart 45-3)

1. Based on your knowledge of PID, you know that the inflammatory condition of the pelvic cavity may involve the following five areas:

    a. _____   d. _____
    b. _____   e. _____
    c. _____

2. Choose six words to describe the characteristics of the infection.

    a. _____   d. _____
    b. _____   e. _____
    c. _____   f. _____

3. The infection is caused by a:

   a. bacteria.

   b. fungus.

   c. parasite.

   d. virus.

4. Name the two most common causative organisms for PID.

   a._____ and   b. _____

5. List four disorders that can result from the PID infection:

   a. _____

   b. _____

   c. _____

   d. _____

6. Name three localized symptoms of PID and six generalized symptoms:

   Localized:

   a. _____   c. _____

   b. _____

   Generalized:

   a. _____   d. _____

   b. _____   e. _____

   c. _____   f. _____

7. Develop a nursing teaching plan for Donna that addresses specific points for avoiding and controlling the illness as well as identifying and managing complications. (Reference pages 1274-1275)

Case Study: Herpes Genitalis

Paige, a 37-year-old mother of one, has just been recently diagnosed with Herpes Genitalis.

1. Herpes Genitalis, a sexually transmitted disease, causes blisters on the:

   a. cervix.

   b. external genitalia.

   c. vagina.

   d. areas all described above.

2. The initial painful infection lasts _____ week(s).

   a. one

   b. two

   c. four

   d. six

3. Choose the herpes virus that is accountable for the majority of genital and perineal lesions:

    a. Epstein-Barr

    b. Cytomegalovirus

    c. Herpes Simplex Type 2

    d. Varicella Zoster.

4. In order to acquire the infection, one must have close human contact by one of five ways. List the five possible ways:

    (a) _____ (b) _____ (c) _____

    (d) _____ and (e) _____ .

5. The virus is killed by: _____ .

6. The antiviral agent that can alter the course of the infection is: _____ .

7. List the nursing diagnoses for Paige:

    a. _____

    b. _____

    c. _____

46

Assessment and Management of Patients with Breast Disorders

I. Learning Objectives:

In addition to the learning objectives on page 1301, I want my students to be able to:

1. _____

2. _____

3. _____

II. Top Terms:

1. Areola
2. BSE
3. Dimpling
4. Fibroadenoma
5. Fibrocystic
6. Galactography

7. Lumpectomy
8. Macromastia
9. Mastitis
10. Menses
11. Paget's Disease
12. Papilloma

III. Collaborative Learning Activities:

Team Discussion Questions/Seminar Topics

1. Explain the significance of the orange-peel appearance (peau d'orange) of breast tissue which is a sign of advanced breast cancer.

2. Discuss the advantage of ultrasound in conjunction with mammography as a way to diagnose breast cancer.

IV. Collaborative Learning Activities:

In-Class Team Exercises

1. Divide the students into several teams. Have each team distinguish between the four stages of breast cancer using the TNM system. Then illustrate an example of each on a drawing of a breast. (reference pages 1310-1313 and Figure 46-4)

2. Complete the following chart for specific chemotherapeutic drugs. (reference pages 1317-1318 and Table 46-4)

Drug Agent	Therapeutic Goal	Side-Effects	Interventions
Adriamycin			
Cytoxan			
5-FU			
DES			
Megace			
Tamoxifen			

Send-Home Assignments

Collect the following information about risk factors for breast cancer by interviewing ten women. Use weighted factors. If risk factor is absent, put a "0" in the box. Summarize the results of your data and try to determine an individual's risk for developing breast cancer. Document any similarities among the women. (reference pages 1310-1311)

Weight Factors	Individual Risk Factors	1	2	3	4	5	6	7	8	9	10
2	Personal History										
4	Genetic History										
1	Early Menarche										
2	Child > 30										
2	Menopause >50										
2	History of Breast Disease										
2	Obesity										
1	Oral Contraceptives										
1	Hormone Therapy										
1	Daily Alcohol										
2	Radiation Exposure										
	TOTAL SCORES:										

47

Assessment and Management of Patients with Disorders of the Male Reproductive System

I. Learning Objectives:

In addition to the learning objectives on page 1335, I want my students to be able to:

1. _____

2. _____

3. _____

II. Top Terms:

1. Benign Prostatic Hyperplasia (BPH)
2. Cowper's Gland
3. Cryosurgery
4. Epididymitis
5. Hydrocele
6. Impotence
7. Orchiectomy
8. Prostate Gland
9. Prostate-Specific Antigen
10. Prostatodynmia
11. Spermatozoa
12. Testosterone

III. Collaborative Learning Activities:

Team Discussion Questions/Seminar Topics

1. Explain, and support with a scientific rationale, the medical management and patient education guidelines for a patient with acute bacterial prostatitis.

2. Explain how and why DES is used for the treatment of prostatectomy.

IV. Critical Thinking Activities:

In-Class Team Exercises

Complete the following chart for the surgical approaches for prostatectomy. (reference page 1342. Table 47-2)

Surgical Approach	Rationale for Choice	Purpose	Pre-Operative Teaching Issues	Post-Operative Education
Transurethral Resection				
Suprapubic Approach				
Perineal Approach				
Retropubic Approach				

Send-Home Assignments

Read the following case study. Fill in the blanks or circle the correct answer.

Case Study: The Patient Undergoing Prostatectomy

Tom is a 65-year-old college administrator who is scheduled for a prostatectomy. (reference pages 1341-1347)

1. Preoperatively, two objectives to determine readiness for surgery are:

   a. _____

   b. _____

2. Prostatectomy must be performed *before*:

3. Choose the most commonly performed surgical procedure that is carried out through endoscopy:

   a. Perinial Approach

   b. Retropubic Approach

   c. Suprapubic Approach

   d. Transurethral Approach

4. List two possible postoperative complications of the TUR approach:

   a.

   b.

5. List four general postoperative complications of a prostatectomy.

   a. _____   c. _____
   b. _____   d. _____

6. Explain why impotence may result from a prostatectomy.

7. Choose three possible preoperative nursing diagnoses:

   a. _____   c. _____
   b. _____

8. Identify two nursing activities to help relieve postoperative bladder spasms:

   a. _____   b. _____

9. Explain why the patient is advised not to sit for prolonged periods of time immediately after surgery.

10. Describe how you would teach a patient to do perineal exercises.

Instructional Improvement Tool for Unit

Student feedback/evaluation indicated that I need to improve my classroom presentation by:

Adding Content

    1. _____

    _____

    2. _____

    _____

    3. _____

    _____

Deleting Content

    1. _____

    _____

    2. _____

    _____

    3. _____

    _____

Emphasizing/De-emphasizing the Following Content

    1. _____

    _____

    2. _____

    _____

    3. _____

    _____

Questions students asked that I need to research for the future are:

    1. _____

    _____

    2. _____

    _____

    3. _____

    _____

48

Assessment of Immune Function

I. Learning Objectives:

In addition to the learning objectives on page 1365, I want my students to be able to:

1. _____

2. _____

3. _____

II. Top Terms:

1. Agglutination
2. Chemotaxis
3. Complement

4. Phagocytosis
5. T-Lymphocytes

III. Collaborative Learning Activities:

Team Discussion Questions/Seminar Topics

1. Explain how pathologic changes occur for three disorders of the immune system: disorders related to autoimmunity, disorders related to hypersensitivity, and disorders related to gammopathies.

2. Design a poster for school children that explains the differences between natural and acquired immunity.

3. Explain how a humoral response to an invading organism results in the production of T-lymphocytes.

IV. Creative Thinking Activities:

In-Class Team Exercises

Consider each of the three variables that significantly influence the body's immunologic response. For each variable explain why it impacts on the immune system. From each rationale, develop a patient teaching guideline to help individuals minimize the variable impact on their body. (reference pages 1375-1376)

Factor Affecting Immune Response	Rationale	Prevention Guidelines
Age		
Gender		
Nutrition		

Send-Home Assignments

Complete the following chart indicating how specific medications cause immunosuppression. For each effect, suggest a patient teaching guideline to help the individual cope with or offset the negative impact of the medication. (reference page 1376, and Table 48-3)

Drug Classification	Effect on Immune System	Patient Teaching Guideline
Antibiotics		
Corticosteroids		
NSAIDs		
Cytotoxic Agents		

49

Management of Patients with Immunodeficiency Disorders

I. Learning Objectives:

In addition to the learning objectives on page 1381, I want my students to be able to:

1. _____

2. _____

3. _____

II. Top Terms:

1. B-Lymphocytes
2. Candidiasis
3. Complement System
4. Cytocidol

5. Gamma Globulin
6. Job's Syndrome
7. Phagocytic Cells
8. T-Lymphocytes

III. Collaborative Learning Activities:

Team Discussion Questions/Seminar Topics

1. Compare the nursing and medical management of patients with primary immunodeficiencies to those with secondary immunodeficiencies.

2. Draft a nursing care plan for a patient receiving intravenous gamma globulin.

3. Choose nursing diagnoses and related nursing interventions for a patient with CVID.

IV. Critical Thinking Activities

In-Class Team Exercises

Read each analogy. Fill in the space provided with the best response. Explain the correlation. (reference pages 1382-1385)

1. Job's Syndrome : phogocytic dysfunction :: Bruton's disease : _____.

2. Colony-stimulating factor : HIE Syndrome :: IV gamma globulin : _____.

3. CVID : Haemophilus influenza :: Ataxia-telangiectasia : _____.

4. DeGeorge's Syndrome : hyperparathyroidism :: chronic mucocutaneous candidiasis : _____ and _____.

5. Angioneurotic edema : frequent episodes of edema :: paroxysmal nocturnal hemoglobinuria : _____.

Send-Home Assignments

For each immunodeficiency disorder, identify its associated immune component, major symptoms, recommended treatments and related patient teaching guidelines (reference page 1383 and Table 49-1)

Immunodeficiency Disorder	Immune Component	Major Symptoms	Treatment	Patient Teaching Guidelines
	Phagocytic Cells			
	B-Lymphocytes			
	T-Lymphocytes			
	B&T Lymphocytes			
	Complement System			

ETHICAL QUESTION: SHOULD ALL PATIENTS BE SCREENED FOR HIV UPON HOSPITAL ADMISSION?

Discussion: The human immunodeficiency virus (HIV) causes AIDS, a still incurable and ultimately fatal disease. Many HIV-positive people are unaware that they carry the virus; this can allow the virus to spread. The virus is spread through blood and body fluids contact, contact which puts health care workers at risk for infection. A policy that would screen all patients for HIV would serve to reduce the spread of the disease and protect the health care workers who care for patients. Would this infringe on the liberty and privacy of patients?

Dilemma: The patient's right to privacy conflicts with health care workers' rights to protection from HIV infection (autonomy versus integrity of the professions). The patient's right to privacy conflicts with society's need to contain the deadly virus and stem a deadly epidemic (autonomy versus justice).

Arguments in FAVOR of screening all patients for HIV: Patients would be informed of their HIV status and, if HIV positive, could seek early treatment for AIDS. The spread of HIV and AIDS could be curbed if patients knew they were positive, knew the importance of changing their high-risk behavior, and notified those whom they may have exposed to HIV. Testing of all hospital patients for HIV would give definitive data on how many patients are HIV positive. Society's need to control the AIDS epidemic is more important than an individual's privacy. Health care workers would know which patients were HIV positive and would take special measures to protect themselves from infection from those patients.

Implications of choosing this position: There would be a very high cost for HIV testing for a very low return in numbers of HIV positive patients. The information that a patient is HIV positive can be devastating to that patient's life, job, housing and health insurance. Patients who thought that they might be HIV positive might avoid necessary health care if they knew they would be tested for HIV. Health care providers may be careless in using precautions against infection with patients testing HIV negative, even though they would still be at risk for hepatitis infection and the patient may have had a falsely negative test.

Arguments AGAINST screening all hospital patients for HIV: A patient's privacy is more important than attempts to stem the spread of AIDS. The high cost of testing is not justified given the relatively low rate of HIV infection. The lack of testing might encourage HIV-positive patients to seek needed medical treatment. Universal precautions should serve to protect health care workers from many known and unknown infectious diseases.

Implications of choosing this position: An opportunity to gather scientific data about the size of the epidemic and to control the spread of the virus would be lost. Health care providers may feel threatened by possible HIV infection from their patients. Patients who are unknowingly HIV positive and remain untested will not learn that information and will not know to seek early treatment for AIDS.

Potential compromise: Seek informed consent for HIV testing for all patients whose history indicates a risk of possible exposure to the virus. Health care providers should use universal precautions in caring for all patients.

Implications of choosing this position: Individual rights are respected, but patients are approached for testing who might otherwise not have been approached. Testing would be haphazard. Some health care workers will only use precautions for those whom they guess to be HIV positive.

Guidelines for the nurse caring for an HIV positive patient:

1. Practice universal precautions as you would for any patient. Avoid labeling the patient in an obvious way (such as by labeling the chart 'AIDS patient,' using more isolation material than is required for the patient, or using ominous warning signs outside the patient's room) so that the lay public and other hospital employees who should not have access to patient information could guess that the patient is HIV positive.

2. Help the patient and professionals distinguish between the HIV virus and the disease of AIDS.

3. Maintain confidentiality of the patient's HIV status.

4. Assess your patient's knowledge level of HIV and AIDS. Initiate teaching plan.

Bibliography

Agency for Health Care Policy and Research (AHCPR) Guidelines: Evaluation and Management of Early HIV Infection. Clinical Practice Guideline, AHCPR Publication No. 94-0572. Rockville, MD: Agency for Health Care Policy and Research, Public Health Service, U.S. Department of Health and Human Services, January, 1994.

American Nurses' Association Committee on Ethics. Statements Regarding Risk versus Responsibility in Providing Nursing Care. Ethics in Nursing: Position Statements and Guidelines. Kansas City, MO, American Nurses' Association, 1988:6-7.

Bayer R. et. al. HIV Antibody Screening: An Ethical Framework for Evaluating Proposed Programs. Journal of the American Medical Association. 1986 October 6; 256(13): 1768-1774.

Freedman B. Health Professions, Codes and the Right to Refuse to Treat HIV-Infectious Patients. Hastings Center Report. 1988 April-May Special Supplement; 18(2): 20-25.

Fox DM. From TB to AIDS: Value Conflicts in Reporting Disease. Hastings Center Report. 1986 December Special Supplement; 16(6): 11-23.

Meritt DJ. The Constitutional Balance Between Health and Liberty. Hastings Center Report. 1986 December Special Supplement: 16(6) 2-10.

Pressures Grow for AIDS Testing; Court Backs Patients' Rights. J Nurs. 1991 June; 91(6): 96,102.

50
Acquired Immunodeficiency Syndrome

I. Learning Objectives:

In addition to the learning objectives on page 1389, I want my students to be able to:

1. _____

2. _____

3. _____

II. Top Terms:

1. Alpha-Interferon
2. Cachexia
3. Karposi's Sarcoma
4. Paresis
5. Pneumocystis carinii pneumonia
6. Retrovir
7. Retrovirus
8. T4 Cells
9. Wasting Syndrome

III. Collaborative Learning Activities:

Team Discussion Questions/Seminar Topics

1. Explain how a permanent infection with HIV is established through altered RNA and DNA.

2. Discuss specific nursing interventions for specific side-effects of the antiretroviral agents: Retrovir, Videx, HIVID, Zerit, and Foscavir.

3. Discuss and give specific examples of how health care providers can maintain "Universal Blood and Body Fluid Precautions" to prevent HIV transmission.

IV. Collaborative Learning Activities:

In-Class Team Exercises

Complete the following chart comparing various laboratory tests with findings related to the diagnosis and tracking of HIV. (reference page 1397, Table 50-1)

HIV Antibody Test	Findings Related to HIV Infection
1. HIV Antibody Tests ELISA IFA RIPA	
2. HIV Tracking PCR PMBC Quantitative Cell Cultures B_2 Microglobulin	
3. Immune Status % CD4 + Cells CD4 : CD8 ratio CD4 cell function tests Immunoglobulin tests Skin Test Sensitivity Reactions	

Send-Home Assignments

Draft a nursing care plan for a 24-year-old single male who has just been diagnosed with AIDS after being admitted to an acute care facility with pneumocystitis carinii pneumonia. The patient is a recent college graduate, employed full-time and engaged to be married in six months. He currently lives at home with his parents and two sisters. (reference pages 1410-1415 and NCP 50-1). Use the following format.

Nursing Dx	Nursing Interventions	Rationale	Expected Outcome

51

Assessment and Management of Patients with Allergic Disorders

I. Learning Objectives:

In addition to the learning objectives on page 1421, I want my students to be able to:

1. _____

2. _____

3. _____

II. Top Terms:

1. Agglutination
2. Allergens
3. Anaphylactoid Reaction
4. Angioedema
5. Antibodies
6. Antigens
7. Bradykinin
8. Epinephrine
9. Histamine
10. Immunoglobulins
11. Lymphokinines
12. Mast Cells
13. Prostaglandins
14. RAST
15. Serotonin
16. T-Cells
17. Urticaria
18. Wheal

III. Collaborative Learning Activities:

Team Discussion Questions/Seminar Topics

1. Discuss the three ways that antibodies are known to react with antigens and give a scientific rationale for each.

2. Explain the difference between actively and passively acquired immunization.

3. Describe how the body responds to specific allergens by releasing common chemical mediators.

IV. Critical Thinking Activities

In-Class Team Exercises

Compare and contrast the etiology, diagnosis, clinical manifestations, medical management and nursing teaching points for the four types of contact dermatitis. (reference pages 1438-1439 and Table 51-4)

Type of Contact Dermatitis	Etiology	Diagnosis	Clinical Manifestations	Medical Management	Nursing Teaching Points
Allergic					
Irritant					
Phototoxic					
Photoallergic					

Send-Home Assignments

Conduct an Allergy Assessment on ten friends or relatives using the Allergy Assessment Sheet from Chart 51-1. After obtaining the data, summarize the results to see if there are any patterns of sensitivity reactions based on seasons, physical agents, habits, geographic area or home location. Also correlate medication use with management.

Allergy Assessment Sheet

Name: _____ Age: ____ Sex ____ Date: _____

I. Chief complaint: _____

II. Present Illness: _____

III. Collateral allergic symptoms: _____

    Eyes: Pruritus _____ Burning _____ Lacrimation _____

                 Swelling _____ Injection _____ Discharge _____

    Ears: Pruritus _____ Fullness _____ Popping _____

                 Frequent infections _____

    Nose: Sneezing _____ Rhinorrhea _____ Obstruction _____

                 Pruritus _____ Mouth-breathing _____

                 Purukent discharge _____

    Throat: Soreness _____ Postnasal discharge _____

                 Palatal pruritus _____ Mucus in the morning _____

    Chest: Cough _____ Pain _____ Wheezing _____

                 Sputum _____ Dyspnea _____

                 Color _____ Rest _____

                 Amount _____ Exertion _____

    Skin: Dermatits _____ Eczema _____ Urticaria _____

IV. Family Allergies

V. Previous allergic treatment or testing: _____

    Prior skin testing: _____

    Medications: Antihistamines   Improved _____ Unimproved _____

                 Bronchodilator   Improved _____ Unimproved _____

                 Nose drops   Improved _____ Unimproved _____

                 Hyposensitization   Improved _____ Unimproved _____

                     Duration _____

                     Antigens _____

                     Reactions _____

                 Antibiotics   Improved _____ Unimproved _____

                 Corticosteroids   Improved _____ Unimproved _____

VI. Physical agents and habits: _____

Bothered by:

Tobacco for _____ years   Alcohol _____   Air Cond. _____

Cigarettes _____ packs/day   Heat _____   Muggy weather _____

Cigars _____ per day   Cold _____   Weather changes _____

Pipes _____ per day   Perfumes _____   Chemicals _____

Never smoked _____   Paints _____   Hair spray _____

Bothered by smoke _____   Insecticides _____   Newspapers _____

                             Cosmetics _____

VII. When symptoms occur: _____

    Time and circumstances of 1st episode: _____

    Prior Health: _____

    Course of illness over decades: progressing _____ regressing _____

    Time of year: _____ Exact dates: _____

        Perennial _____

        Seasonal _____

        Seasonally exacerbated _____

    Monthly variations (menses, occupation): _____

    Time of week (weekends vs. weekdays): _____

    Time of day or night: _____

    After insect stings: _____

VIII. Where symptoms occur: _____

    Living where at onset: _____

    Living where since onset: _____

    Effect of vacation or major geographic change: _____

    Symptoms better indoors or outdoors: _____

    Effect of school or work: _____

    Effect of staying elsewhere nearby: _____

    Effect of hospitalization: _____

    Effect of specific environments: _____

    Do symptoms occur around: _____

        old leaves _____ hay _____ lakeside _____ barns _____

        summer homes _____ damp basement _____ dry attic _____

        lawnmowing _____ animals _____ other _____

    Do symptoms occur after eating: _____

        cheese _____ mushrooms _____ beer _____ melons _____

        bananas _____ fish _____ nuts _____ citrus fruits _____

    Home: city _____ rural _____

            house _____ age _____

            apartment _____ basement _____ damp _____ dry _____

            heating sytem _____

            pets (how long) _____ dog _____ cat _____ other _____

Bedroom:	Type	Age	*Living room*:	Type	Age
Pillow	____	____	Rug	____	____
Mattress	____	____	Matting	____	____
Blankets	____	____	Furniture	____	____
Quilts	____	____			
Furniture	____	____			

    Anywhere in home symptoms are worse? _____

IX. What does patient think makes symptoms worse? _____

X. Under what circumstances is patient free of symptoms? _____

XI. Summary and additional comments: _____

52

Management of Patients with Rheumatic Disorders

I. Learning Objectives:

In addition to the learning objectives on page 1443, I want my students to be able to:

1. _____

2. _____

3. _____

II. Top Terms:

1. Arthrography
2. Diarthrodial
3. Exacerbation
4. Fibromyalgia
5. Hemarthrosis
6. Osteopenia
7. Osteophytes
8. Pannus
9. Remission
10. Scleroderma
11. Synovial

III. Collaborative Learning Activities:

Team Discussion Questions/Seminar Topics

1. Compare and contrast the etiology, clinical manifestations and medical management for the three types of lupus erythematosus: discoid, systemic, and drug-induced.

2. Describe several common undesirable side-effects of corticosteroid therapy and list a nursing intervention for each side-effect.

IV. Collaborative Learning Activities:

In-Class Team Exercises

Match the clinical interpretation/laboratory significance listed in Column II with its associated test listed in Column I. (reference pages 4150-1451, Table 52-1).

Column I		Column II	
___	1. Uric Acid	a.	decrease can be seen in chronic inflammation
___	2. Complement	b.	this positive test is associated with SLE, RA, and Raynaud's disease
___	3. Rheumatoid Factor	c.	an increase in this substance is seen with gout
___	4. Hematocrit	d.	this protein substance decreased in RA and SLE
___	5. HLA-B27 Antigen	e.	this is present in 80% of those who have rheumatoid arthritis
___	6. Antinuclear Antibody (ANA)	f.	this is present in 85% of those with ankylosing spondylitis

Match the classification of rheumatic diseases listed in Column II with its associated specific disease listed in Column I. An answer may be used more than once. (reference page 1444, Chart 52-1)

Column I		Column II	
___	1. Carpal Tunnel Syndrome	a.	Diffuse Connective Tissue Disorder
___	2. Osteoporosis and Osteomalacia	b.	Extraarticular Disorders
___	3. Scleroderma	c.	Neurovascular Disorders
___	4. Psoriatic Arthritis	d.	Bone and Cartilage Disorders
___	5. Epicondylitis	e.	Spondyloarthropathies
___	6. Multiple Myeloma	f.	Metabolic and Endocrine Disease
___	7. Raynaud's Phenomenon	g.	Neoplasms
___	8. Acromegaly		
___	9. Reiter's Syndrome		
___	10. Paget's Disease		

Review Figure 52-1 which depicts the results of the inflammatory response in the knee joint. Outline, in detail, the series of related steps that lead to the inflammation beginning with the antigen stimulus that activates monocytes and T-Lumphocytes (reference page 1445)

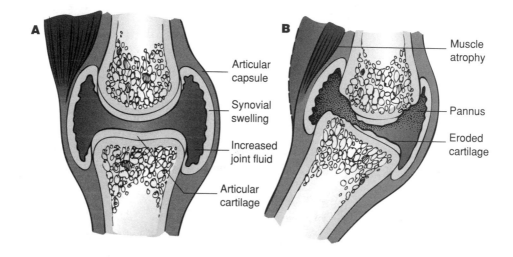

Instructional Improvement Tool for Unit

Student feedback/evaluation indicated that I need to improve my classroom presentation by:

Adding Content

1. _____

   _____

2. _____

   _____

3. _____

   _____

Deleting Content

1. _____

   _____

2. _____

   _____

3. _____

   _____

Emphasizing/De emphasizing the Following Content

1. _____

   _____

2. _____

   _____

3. _____

   _____

Questions students asked that I need to research for the future are:

1. _____

   _____

2. _____

   _____

3. _____

   _____

53

Assessment of Integumentary Function

I. Learning Objectives:

In addition to the learning objectives on page 1477, I want my students to be able to:

1. _____

2. _____

3. _____

II. Top Terms:

1. Beau's Lines
2. Cutaneous
3. Ecchymosis
4. Insensible Perspiration
5. Keratin
6. Melanin

7. Pruritus
8. Purpura Petechia
9. Sebaceous Glands
10. Telangiectasis
11. Turgor

III. Collaborative Learning Activities:

Team Discussion Questions/Seminar Topics

1. Compare and contrast the functions of the three layers of skin: epidermis, dermis, and the subcutaneous tissues.

2. Distinguish between primary and secondary skin lesions and give three examples of each. For each, describe the lesion's characteristics that aid in diagnosis.

3. Describe the six common examples of nail disorders. Examine some of your classmates' nails and determine if you can find other examples not listed in Figure 53-7.

IV. Critical Thinking Activities:

In-Class Team Exercises

Separate students into several teams. Have each team conduct a patient history on one member who has or "pretends" to have a skin disorder. Have each team record their findings and come to a diagnosis. Then each team needs to share their clusters of data and ask other teams to identify the skin disorder. Use Chart 53-1 below for the outline of interview/assessment questions.

CHART 53-1
Patient History: Skin Disorders

Patient history relevant to skin disorders may be obtained by asking the following questions:

- When did you first notice this skin problem (also investigate duration and intensity)?
- Has it occurred previously?
- Are there any other symptoms?
- What site was first affected?
- What did the rash or lesion look like when it first appeared?
- Where and how fast did it spread?
- Are there itching, burning, tingling, or crawling sensations?
- Is there any loss of sensation?
- Is the problem worse at a particular time or season?
- Do you have any idea how it started?
- Do you have a history of hay fever, asthma, hives, eczema, or allergies?
- Does anyone in your family have skin problems or rashes?
- Did the eruptions appear after certain foods were eaten?
- Had there been recent intake of alcohol?
- Was there a relation between a specific event and the outbreak of the rash or lesion?
- What medications are you taking?
- What topical medication (ointment, cream, salve) have you put on the lesion (include over-the-counter medications)?
- What skin products or cosmetics do you use?
- What is your occupation?
- What in your immediate environment (plants, animals, chemicals, infections) might be precipitating this problem? Is there anything new or are there any changes in the environment?
- Does anything touching your skin cause a rash?
- Is there anything else you wish to talk about in regard to this problem?

Send-Home Assignments

Match the descriptions of specific skin lesions listed in Column II with their associated type listed in Column I. (reference pages 1486-1488 [Chart 53-2])

Part I

Column I

_____ 1. bulla

_____ 2. crusts

_____ 3. macule

_____ 4. nodule

_____ 5. wheal

Column II

a. a covering formed from serum, blood, or pus drying on the skin

b. a large vesicle or blister greater than 1 cm in diameter

c. a nonelevated discoloration of the skin

d. a raised solid lesion larger than 1 cm in diameter

e. a transient elevation of the skin caused by edema of the dermis and capillary dilatation

Part II

_____ 1. papule

_____ 2. plaque

_____ 3. pustule

_____ 4. scales

_____ 5. vesicle

a. a lesion that contains pus, i.e., acne

b. a small elevation of the skin that is filled with clear fluid

c. a solid elevated lesion on the skin or mucous membrane that is greater than 1 cm in diameter

d. a solid elevated palpable lesion that is less than 1 cm in diameter

e. heaped-up horny layers of dead epidermis

54
Management of Patients with Dermatologic Problems

I. Learning Objectives:

In addition to the learning objectives on page 1493, I want my students to be able to:

1. _____

2. _____

3. _____

II. Top Terms:

1. Alopecia
2. Argon Laser
3. Comedones
4. Cryosurgery
5. Dermabrasion
6. Granular Tissue
7. Hematopoietic
8. Keloids
9. Keratoses
10. Lichenification
11. Melanoma
12. Pedicle Flap
13. Rhytidectomy
14. Seborrhea
15. Sebum
16. Xerosis

III. Collaborative Learning Activities:

Team Discussion Questions/Seminar Topics

1. Explain why the herpes zoster virus is becoming more prevalent in individuals who are immunocompromised.

2. Compare and contrast the etiology, clinical manifestations, diagnostic evaluation, and medical management of basal cell and squamous cell carcinoma.

IV. Critical Thinking Activities

In-Class Team Exercises

1. Design a poster outlining patient education needs for those with infections of the skin. (reference pages 1509-1511)

2. Complete the following chart comparing the five types of tinea infections. (reference pages 1511-1513, Table 54-5)

Tinea Infection	Location	Clinical Manifestations	Medical Treatment	Patient Care Education
Tinea Capitis				
Tinea Corporis				
Tinea Cruris				
Tinea Pedis				
Tinea Unguium				

Send-Home Assignments

Read the following case study. Fill in the blanks or circle the correct answer.

Case Study: Acne Vulgaris

Brian is a 15-year-old who has been experiencing facial eruptions of acne for about a year. The numerous lesions are inflamed and present on the face and neck. He has tried many over-the-counter medications and nothing seems to help. His father had a history of severe acne when he was a teenager. (reference pages 1505-1509)

1. Based on your knowledge of acne vulgaris, you know that the skin disorder is characterized by five types of lesions:
   (a) _____, (b) _____, (c) _____,
   (d) _____, and (e) _____.

2. The etiology of acne stems from:

   a. genetic factors.

   b. hormonal factors.

   c. bacterial factors.

   d. an interplay of all of the above.

3. Acne, most prevalent at puberty, is the direct result of oversecretion of the _____ glands.

   a. exocrine

   b. lacrimal

   c. sebaceous

   d. mucous

4. Explain the rationale for using Benzoyl Peroxide:

   _____

5. Explain the rationale for using Vitamin A Acid:

   _____

6. Choose a common antibiotic that is frequently prescribed for the treatment of acne:

   a. terbutaline

   b. tamoxifen

   c. tetracycline

   d. terfenadine

7. Choose the common oral retinoid that is used for acne:

    a. Accutane

    b. Acne-Aid

    c. Actinex

    d. Adalat

8. Based on assessment data, identify two collaborative problems:

    (a) _____ and (b) _____

55

Management of Patients with Burn Injury

I. Learning Objectives:

In addition to the learning objectives on page 1545, I want my students to be able to:

1. _____

2. _____

3. _____

II. Top Terms:

1. Biobane
2. Colloids
3. Compartment Syndrome
4. Crystalloids
5. Debridement
6. Escharotomy

7. Hypothermia
8. Interstitial Fluid
9. Ischemia
10. Keloid
11. Paralytic Ileus
12. Partial-Thickness Burns

III. Collaborative Learning Activities:

Team Discussion Questions/Seminar Topics

1. Compare and contrast the causes and resultant physiological responses between the three categories of pulmonary burn injuries.

2. Explain exactly why carbon monoxide inhalation injuries are so fatal.

3. Describe the rationale behind the criteria for adequate burn injury treatment: systolic BP > 100 mg Hg, HR < 110/min., and urine output > 30 ml/hr.

IV. Critical Thinking Exercises:

In-Class Team Exercises

Complete the following chart comparing the characteristics of the three classifications of burns. (reference pages 1549-1550 and Table 55-1)

Burn Classification	Layer of Skin Involved	Possible Cause	Clinical Manifestations	Treatment
Superficial (First-Degree)				
Partial-Thickness (Second-Degree)				
Full-Thickness (Third Degree)				

Send-Home Assignments

Complete the following flow chart illustrating the pathophysiological sequence of reactions that result from a systemic response to a burn injury. (reference pages 1546-1549)

Flow Chart: Systemic Response to Burn Injury

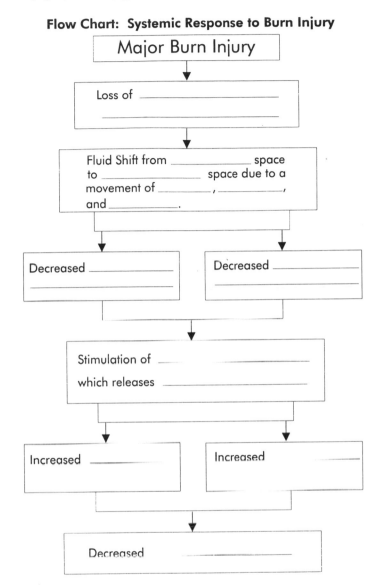

ETHICAL QUESTION: CAN CHILDREN REFUSE PAINFUL BURN TREATMENT?

Discussion: Household accidents often result in burns of children. The treatment and recovery from burns can be long and painful, and it requires the cooperation of the patient. Adults have the right to refuse this treatment if they find that the burdens of the treatment outweigh the benefits. Should children be allowed to refuse treatment? How old should a child be before health care professionals take their views seriously? If a seventeen year old youth wants to refuse treatment and his parents want the treatment to continue, who should prevail?

Dilemma: The minor's desire to refuse treatment conflicts with the parents' and health care professionals' obligation to do what is best for the patient (autonomy versus beneficence).

Arguments that children SHOULD be allowed to refuse painful treatment: Children can understand risks and benefits of treatment, which is the major component of competency. Autonomy is more important than beneficence.

Implication of choosing this position: Children may die if treatment is abandoned prematurely for impulsive reasons. Health care professionals may feel guilty if the patient's treatment is abandoned prematurely. There is a possibility that legal proceedings would need to take place to declare the patient competent to make medical decisions.

Arguments that children SHOULD NOT be allowed to refuse treatment: Children can only see the here-and-now discomfort of burn treatment and cannot understand long range goals. They cannot properly evaluate the risks and benefits of treatment and therefore are not competent. Decisions for minors should be made on a "best interests" (beneficence) basis and not on a child's views.

Implications of choosing this position: Children will suffer because of treatment. The cooperation of the child with treatment may be more difficult to obtain if the child has no say in his care. Health care professionals may feel guilty about treating a patient against his will. Professionals and parents may feel guilty if the patient dies after treatment given against his will.

Potential Compromise: Evaluate the child's refusal of treatment on a case-by-case basis. Assess the child's ability to weigh benefits and burdens of treatment and proceed with measures to discuss stopping treatment for children able to articulate coherent reasons for doing so.

Implications of this position: This position upholds respect for the autonomy of children who are able to communicate an understanding of the burdens and benefits of treatment, but it may threaten or upset the parents of children for whom legal proceedings are being pursued.

Guidelines for the nurse caring for a child who wants painful treatment stopped:

1. Review the chart for patient's age, history, cause of burn, course of burn treatment, family and social situation, current treatment burdens, goals of treatment and expected outcomes.

2. Discuss the treatment with the patient. Discover the concerns, level of maturity and understanding of treatment and document them. Assess if the patient's refusal stems from part of the plan of care that can be adjusted, for example, pain control that is inadequate.

3. Discuss the matter with the patient's physicians. Consider alternative treatment measures that might make the treatment more palatable to the patient.

4. Develop creative nursing measures that will increase the patient's level of control and decrease pain.

5. Seek parental support of the treatment plan and involve them in the plan of care. Consider social work, chaplain, and psychiatric nurse consultations if they are appropriate and not already in place.

6. Institute a patient care conference if the patient continues to refuse treatment. Include all family and health care providers involved in the patient's case.

7. If the child is older, shows good understanding of risks and benefits of treatment, and can verbalize a coherent reason for refusing treatment, consult with the bioethics committee.

Bibliography

Deatrick JA. et. al. Children Should be Seen and Heard: Chronically Ill Children Should have a Voice in Treatment Decisions. Health Progress. 1990 April:76-79.

King NMP and Cross AW. Children as Decision-Makers: Guidelines for Pediatricians. Journal of Pediatrics. 1989 July; 115(l):10-16.

Leikin S. A Proposal Concerning Decisions to Forgo Life-Sustaining Treatment for Young People. Journal of Pediatrics. 1989 July; 115(l):17-22.

Instructional Improvement Tool for Unit

Student feedback/evaluation indicated that I need to improve my classroom presentation by:

Adding Content

1. _____
   _____
2. _____
   _____
3. _____
   _____

Deleting Content

1. _____
   _____
2. _____
   _____
3. _____
   _____

Emphasizing/De-emphasizing the Following Content

1. _____
   _____
2. _____
   _____
3. _____
   _____

Questions students asked that I need to research for the future are:

1. _____
   _____
   _____
2. _____
   _____
3. _____
   _____

56

Assessment and Management of Patients with Vision Problems and Eye Disorders

I. Learning Objectives:

In addition to the learning objectives on page 1587, I want my students to be able to:

1. _____

2. _____

3. _____

II. Top Terms:

1.	Astigmatism	9.	Keratitis
2.	Blepharitis	10.	Myopia
3.	Cataract	11.	Nystagmus
4.	Conjunctiva	12.	Papilledema
5.	Diplopia	13.	Photophobia
6.	Exophthalmus	14.	Ptosis
7.	Glaucoma	15.	Refraction
8.	Hordeolum	16.	Tonometry

III. Collaborative Learning Activities:

Team Discussion Questions/Seminar Topics

1. Compare and contrast the structure and function of the cornea and iris.

2. Provide the physiological reason why night vision is compromised in the elderly.

3. Explain the purpose and process of phacoemulsification for cataract surgery.

4. Explain why the following three conditions are contraindications for intraocular lens (IOL) implants: recurrent uveitis, proliferative diabetic retinopathy, and neovascular glaucoma.

5. Describe the proper procedure for instilling eye drops and applying an ointment to the eyes.

IV. Critical Thinking Activities:

In-Class Team Exercises

1. Have a student bring the Snellen chart into class. Assign students to work in groups and assess each other's visual acuity. Record the acuity readings (i.e., 20/20) on the following chart along with each student's age and any other related conditions (corrective lens use, chronic illnesses, medications). Determine if there is a mean (average) acuity score for the class, per age group, etc. (reference pages 1596-1598)

Student #	Acuity Reading	Corrective Lens	Illness	Medications
1				
2				
3				
4				
5				
6				
7				
8				
9				
10				
11				
12				
13				
14				
15				
16				
17				
18				
19				
20				

2. List one advantage and two disadvantages for each of four types of corrective lenses. (reference pages 1604-1607 and Table 56-1)

Type of Lens	Advantages	Disadvantages
Hard Contact Lenses	1. _____	1. _____ 2. _____
Soft Contact Lenses	1. _____	1. _____ 2. _____
Extended-Wear Lenses	1. _____	1. _____ 2. _____
Progressive-Power Lenses	1. _____	1. _____ 2. _____

Send-Home Assignments

Read the following case study. Fill in the blanks or circle the correct answer.

Case Study: Cataract Surgery

Marcella is a 75-year-old single woman who has had progressive diminished visual acuity and increased difficulty with night driving. Her physician suspects that Marcella has a cataract. He does a complete eye examination and history. (reference pages 93-107 and Chart 56-3)

1. As part of an oral history, the physician tries to determine if Marcella has any of the common factors that contribute to cataract development such as (a) _____, (b) _____, (c) _____, and (d) _____.

2. Marcella, during her history, told the physician that she was experiencing the three common symptoms found with cataracts: (a) _____, (b) _____, and (c) _____.

3. On ophthalmic examination, the physician noted the major objective finding seen with cataracts:

    _____

4. When assessing the need for surgery, the physician determined that Marcella's best corrected vision was worse than the minimal standard of:

    a. 20/15.

    b. 20/25.

    c. 20/35.

    d. 20/50.

5. The physician decided to perform _____, the most preferred technique for cataract surgery.

6. The physician advises Marcella that there is a 25% chance that she may experience the common complication of:

    a. glaucoma.

    b. uveitis.

    c. secondary membranes.

    d. choroidal detachment.

7. Postoperatively, Marcella knows that she will need to wear an eye shield at night for about:

    a. 3 evenings.

    b. one week.

    c. two weeks.

    d. one month.

57

Assessment and Management of Patients with Hearing Problems and Ear Disorders

I. Learning Objectives:

In addition to the learning objectives on page 1643, I want my students to be able to:

1. _____

2. _____

3. _____

II. Top Terms:

1. Audiologist
2. Cerumen
3. Cholesteatoma
4. Cochlea
5. Eustachian Tube
6. Labyrinth
7. Meniere's Disease
8. Organ of Corti
9. Otalgia
10. Otolaryngologist
11. Ototoxicity
12. Presbycusis
13. Proprioceptive System
14. Temporomandibular
15. Tinnitus
16. Tympanic Membrane
17. Vertigo

III. Collaborative Learning Activities:

Send-Home Assignments

1. Compare and contrast how each of the following symptoms reflect problems of the external, middle and inner ear: vertigo, tinnitus, pain, hearing loss and discharge.

2. Compare and contrast the various types of hearing aids relative to advantages, disadvantages, and range of hearing loss.

IV. Critical Thinking Activities:

Team Discussion Questions/Seminar Topics

Read the sentence that defines/explains the scrambled word. Unscramble the word. (reference pages 1644-1646 [Chart 57-1])

1. | A | H | O | C | E | L | C |

A major organ of hearing

2. | L | I | U | S | R | R | C |

Aids in collecting sound waves and passing them onto the auditory canal

3. | E | U | E | C | R | M | N |

Another name for ear wax

4. | S | E | L | M | U | A | L |

An auditory ossicle also known as the "hammer"

5. | S | C | I | U | N |

The middle ossicle, also known as the anvil

6. | H | H | I | E | G | T |

The cranial nerve also known as the cochleovestibular nerve

7. | H | N | R | B | L | A | Y | I | T |

Another word for the vestibular system

8. | C | N | P | Y | T | M | A | I |

This membrane vibrates and transmits sound

Send-Home Assignments

Develop a nursing care plan for Julia, who is 67-years-old, lives alone, and has just been diagnosed as having Meniere's disease. She will be medically managed for her symptoms. Use the following format for development of your care plan. (reference pages 1660-1663)

Nursing Diagnosis:

Immediate Goal(s):

Intermediate Goal(s):

Long-Term Goal(s):

Nursing Interventions   Expected Outcomes

Instructional Improvement Tool for Unit

Student feedback/evaluation indicated that I need to improve my classroom presentation by:

Adding Content

1. _____

_____

2. _____

_____

3. _____

_____

Deleting Content

1. _____

_____

2. _____

_____

3. _____

_____

Emphasizing/De-emphasizing the Following Content

1. _____

_____

2. _____

_____

3. _____

_____

Questions students asked that I need to research for the future are:

1. _____

_____

2. _____

_____

3. _____

_____

58

Assessment of Neurologic Function

I. Learning Objectives:

In addition to the learning objectives on page 1675, I want my students to be able to:

1. _____

2. _____

3. _____

II. Top Terms:

1. Aphasia
2. Ataxia
3. Babinski Reflex
4. Cortical Blindness
5. Dysarthria
6. Dyskinesias
7. Extrapyramidal System
8. Meninges
9. Paraplegia
10. Paresis
11. Ptosis
12. Tinnitus

III. Collaborative Learning Activities:

Team Discussion Questions/Seminar Topics

1. Explain the concept of the "blood-brain barrier" and what it means relative to pharmacotherapy.

2. Demonstrate the Romberg Test, explain the rationale for its use and interpret the results of several possible abnormal outcomes.

3. Explain the purpose, process and interpretation of a negative and positive Babinski response.

4. Distinguish between the terms, delirium and dementia.

IV. Critical Thinking Activities

In-Class Team Exercises

Cranial Nerve Examination

Assign students to groups of four. Each student in every group should have an opportunity to conduct a cranial nerve examination on another student. For each of the following 12 nerves, have a student document the process and the result of the clinical examination. Allot some time at the end of class for the group to share results being sensitive to any abnormalities that might embarrass a student. (reference page 1692, Table 58-2)

Cranial Nerve	Clinical Exam Process	Results and Interpretation
1. Olfactory		
2. Optic		
3. Oculomotor		
4. Trachlear		
5. Trigeminal		
6. Abducens		
7. Facial		
8. Vestibulo-cochlear		
9. Glossopharyngeal		
10. Vagus		
11. Spinal Accessory		
12. Hypoglossal		

Neurological Examination

Using the following outline, complete a neurologic examination on a relative or friend. Compare your results against the expected normal results in the textbook. (reference pages 1687-1695)

Neurologic Examination	Nursing Assessment	Results	Clinical Interpretation
1. **Cerebral Function** Mental Status Thought Process Emotional Status Perception Motor Ability Language Ability Glascow Coma Scale (ref. page 1690, Chart 58-4)			
2. **Cranial Nerves** (use form on previous pages)			
3. **Motor System** Muscle Strength Motor Power Balance & Coordination The Romberg Test			
4. **Reflexes** Biceps Triceps Brachioradialis Patellar Ankle Clonus Abdominal Babinski			
5. **Sensory System** Tactile Pain & Temperature Vibration & Proprioception Position Taste & Smell Tactile & Visual			

59

Management of Patients with Neurologic Dysfunction

I. Learning Objectives:

In addition to the learning objectives on page 1705, I want my students to be able to:

1. _____

2. _____

3. _____

II. Top Terms:

1. Aphasia
2. Craniotomy
3. Decerebration
4. Decortication

5. Diabetes Insipidus
6. Guillain-Barré Syndrome
7. Myasthenia Gravis
8. Weaning

III. Collaborative Learning Activities:

Team Discussion Questions/Seminar Topics

1. Distinguish between the clinical manifestations of stupor and coma, citing the rationale for the differences in each.

2. Divide the students into sub-groups of four. Have each group create a different profile of an aphasic patient. Then have groups trade profiles. After a traded profile is received, each group is to draft up several specific "how-to's" regarding communication with their aphasic patient.

IV. Collaborative Learning Activities:

In-Class Team Exercises

Complete the following chart by documenting specific nursing interventions for a patient with increased ICP. (reference pages 1709-1715 and Table 59-1)

Factor Contributing to ICP	Medical Intervention	Rationale	Nursing Intervention	Patient Education

Send-Home Assignments

Develop a nursing care plan for Mr. Douval, who is 61-years-old and suffering with nonfluent aphasia. He had a stroke about 1 week ago. He lives with his wife and has a strong family support system. (reference pages 1735-1736)

Nursing Diagnosis:

Immediate Goal(s):

Intermediate Goal(s):

Long-Term Goal(s):

Nursing Interventions   Expected Outcomes

Construct a list of preoperative nursing interventions and postoperative nursing interventions (with supporting rationales) for a 57-year-old lawyer who is to undergo intracranial surgery for a brain tumor. He lives in a center city townhouse with his wife, who is also a lawyer. (reference pages 1737-1745 and Chart 59-5)

Nursing Interventions   Rationale

Preoperative Care

Postoperative Care

ETHICAL QUESTION: SHOULD PATIENTS IN A PERSISTENT VEGETATIVE STATE BE USED AS ORGAN DONORS?

Discussion: The need for donated organs for transplantation has long outstripped the supply of organs from brain dead donors. Many more patients fulfill the criteria for persistent vegetative state (PVS) than the criteria for brain death, and the recovery from a PVS is thought to be less than one percent. Many people equate the loss of higher brain functions (thought and perception) with the loss of what is essential to being human. Can the definition of death be changed to include the PVS and then free up the families of those patients to donate their organs?

Dilemma: Obligation to do what is best for the patient conflicts with the needs of the population as a whole (beneficence versus justice).

Arguments in FAVOR of using PVS patients as organ donors: The loss of higher brain function is equivalent to the loss of the human being; therefore the PVS patient should be classified as "dead" just as brain dead patients are classified as "dead." PVS is relatively easy to diagnose and distinguish from other conditions; therefore only PVS patients will be considered as organ donors. The recovery from a PVS is thought to be less than one percent. The needs of many sick people for organs justify changing the current definition of death. It is very costly to maintain PVS patients on artificial nutrition in nursing homes; using PVS patients as organ donors would decrease that number, save money, and provide a source for organs for those in urgent need of them.

Implications for choosing this position: More organs would become available for transplant, which would help many patients on the waiting list for organs, patients who could recover from their disease with the organ transplants and contribute to society. The change in the concept of death from whole brain death to PVS would cause confusion as to what constitutes death. For example, if a spontaneously-breathing, eyes-open moving patient is considered dead, why not an elderly nursing home patient with advanced Alzheimer's Disease? This movement from the intended change in practice to the unanticipated, unintended result is called, in ethical terms, the slippery slope effect.

Arguments AGAINST using PVS patients as organ donors: The small chance of recovery from a PVS is enough to exclude the PVS patient from the category of the dead (the chance of recovery from properly diagnosed brain death is zero). The diagnosis of PVS is not as precise as that of brain death. Not everyone agrees that the loss of higher brain function is equivalent to the loss of human being. PVS patients are people, too. PVS patients should be treated as ends and not as means to an end. The definition of death should remain restricted and tight to avoid initiating the slippery slope effect. This position is consistent with current U.S. law.

Implications of choosing this position: Organs for transplant will remain scarce. The concept of death will not change. Many people who consider PVS patients dead will consider it a waste of organs to either maintain PVS patients on tube feedings or to allow them to die without using their organs.

Guidelines for the nurse caring for a PVS Patient:

1. Review the chart for the patient's history, reason for admission, cause of PVS state, length of PVS state, current treatment and treatment goals. See if any advance directives from the patient are included. Compare the current treatment with that specified in the advances directive.

2. Provide emotional support for the family. Consider psychiatric nurse, social work, chaplaincy consultations for them as appropriate.

3. Discuss the plan of care with the patient's physician. If the current treatment differs from that specified in the advanced directive, explore the reason for this with the physician and consult the bioethics committee if necessary.

4. Does the patient have a DNR order? If not,. why not? Has this issue been explored with the family? Have they refused a DNR order? Why? Plan a patient care conference if needed to facilitate an agreement about a plan of care for the patient among the physician, family, and nursing staff.

5. If the family wants to donate the patient's organs, explain the difference between brain death and PVS. Explain that current U. S. Law forbids the donation of PVS patient organs. Refer them to the physician or the local organ transplant organization if more information is desired.

Bibliography

Armstrong PW. and Colen BD. From Quinlan to Jobes: The Courts and the PVS Patient. Hastings Center Report. 1988 February-March; 18(l): 37-40.

Brody BA. Ethical Questions Raised by the Persistent Vegetative Patient. Hastings Center Report. 1988 February-March; 18(l): 33-37.

Chabalewski F and Norris MKG. The gift of life: Talking to families about organ and tissue donation. Am J Nurs 1994 June; 94(6): 28-33.

Cranford RE. The Persistent Vegetative State: The Medical Reality (Getting the Facts Straight). Hastings Center Report. 1 938 February-March; 18(1): 27-32.

Meilaender G. Terra es animate: On Having a Life. Hastings Center Report. 1993 July-August; 23(4): 25-32.

Schneiderman LJ. Exile and PVS. Hastings Center Report. 1990 May-June; 20(3):5

Steinbock B. Recovery from Persistent Vegetative State?: The Case of Connie Coons. Hastings Center Report 1989 July-August: 19(4) 14-15.

Veatch RM. The Impending Collapse of the Whole-Brain Definition of Death. Hastings Center Report. 1993 July-August.: 23(4): 18-24.

Wikler D. Not Dead, Not Dying? Ethical Categories and Persistent Vegetative State. Hastings Center Report. 1988 February-March; 18(l): 41-47.

Wilke JC. and Andrusko D. Personhood Redux. Hastings Center Report. 1988 October-November; 18(5): 30-33.

Youngner SJ. Human Death and High Technology: The Failure of the Whole-Brain Formulations. Annals of Internal Medicine. 1983 August; 99(2): 252-258.

60

Management of Patients with Neurologic Disorders

I. Learning Objectives:

In addition to the learning objectives on page 1751, I want my students to be able to:

1. _____

2. _____

3. _____

II. Top Terms:

1. Akathisia
2. Ataxia
3. Bradykinesia
4. Cachexia
5. Cephalgia
6. Chorea
7. Glioma

8. Laminectomy
9. Migraine
10. Myelin
11. Papilledema
12. Ptosis
13. Sciatica
14. Status Epilepticus

III. Collaborative Learning Activities:

Team Discussion Questions/Seminar Topics

1. Compare and contrast the different medications and treatment modalities for the various types of migraine headaches.

2. Describe the etiology, pathophysiology, medical management, and nursing intervention for a patient with myasthenia gravis.

3. With another classmate, demonstrate how a spinal cord injury patient should be immobilized at the scene of an accident.

IV. Critical Thinking Activities

In-Class Team Exercises

For each of the following spinal cord injuries, describe the area of cord damage in the brain, the resulting cord syndrome characteristics, and implications for immediate nursing intervention. (reference pages 1796-1800 and Chart 60-8)

Spinal Cord Injury Syndrome	Area of Damage	Cord Syndrome Characteristics	Nursing Interventions
Central Cord			
Anterior Cord			
Lateral Cord			
Complete Lesion			

Send-Home Assignments

Develop an assessment guide for Edward, a 24-year-old who was admitted unconscious to the emergency department with a head injury sustained in a vehicular accident. Share your guide with your classmates for their comments. (reference pages 1788-1790)

After developing your assessment guide for Edward, construct a nursing care plan that will emphasize the following areas: fluid and electrolyte replacement, nutritional management, restlessness, potential complications, and family education. Edward is the adopted son of a couple who are now both retired from schoolteaching. Use the format below and share it with your instructor for comment. (reference pages 1792-1796)

Nursing Diagnosis:

Immediate Goal(s):

Intermediate Goal(s):

Long-Term Goal(s):

Nursing Interventions   **Expected Outcomes**

ETHICAL QUESTION: WHEN SHOULD LIFE-SUPPORT BE DISCONTINUED FROM BRAIN DEAD PATIENTS?

Discussion: Brain death is legally considered a definition of death in all 50 states, but families and health care professionals continue to have difficulty with the concept. As a result, physicians may offer the families of brain dead patients the option to discontinue life support, or they may leave the impression that the brain dead patient might recover. Brain dead patients may be left on life-support for days or even weeks, costing huge amounts of money to support dead patients. Should families be encouraged to agree to the discontinuation of life support for their brain dead family member?

Dilemma: The family's desire to act in the best interests of the patient conflicts with current medical practice (beneficence versus integrity of the health professions).

Arguments in favor of discontinuing life supports for brain dead patients within hours of diagnosis regardless of family wishes: This will prevent a waste of time and resources by limiting the amount of time a brain dead patient is maintained on life-support in the ICU. The quick turnaround time from diagnoses to discontinuance of life-supports will force the family to come to terms with the fact that the patient is dead and prevent the loss of days and weeks if the family is allowed to "think about" turning off life support on a brain dead patient.

Implications of choosing this position: Hospital resources will not be wasted in maintaining brain dead patients on life support. Families may become upset and angry if forced into a pre-arranged timetable for discontinuing life support.

Arguments for waiting for family consent to discontinue life support: This will allow the patient's family to come to terms with the patient's death. Families will not become angry if allowed control over the patient's fate.

Implications of choosing this position: Families may repeatedly delay the withdrawal of life supports for days or weeks, which will waste expensive and often scarce resources. Grieving, distraught families may still become angry at health care workers.

Potential compromise: Emphasize to the family of a brain dead patient that brain death is death and that life-support must and will be discontinued. Work with the family to set a reasonable time at which to discontinue life support; within 24 hours of the determination of brain death is reasonable.

Implication of choosing this position: This allows for some control by the family and allows for some time for family grief work, but still expedites discontinuation of expensive and scarce resources. Families may still become angry at being pressured to agree to the withdrawal of life-support.

Guidelines for the nurse caring for a brain dead patient:

1. Review the patient's chart and note the patient's history, cause of brain death, documentation of brain death, family situation and presence of advance directive from the patient. Assure yourself that brain death documentation has been completed in accordance with hospital policy and state law.

2. Provide emotional support for the family. Initiate psychiatric nurse, social work or chaplaincy consultations for the family as appropriate.

3. Provide teaching and counseling for the family about brain death. Emphasize that brain death **is** death. Distinguish brain death from coma or a persistent vegetative state.

4. In accordance with the physician, consult the local transplant organization about approaching the family regarding the donation of the patient's organs. Federal law requires that families be asked about organ donation. Support the family's decision about organ donation.

5. If the family elects not to donate the patient's organs, encourage the physician to talk with the family regarding the discontinuance of life support. Try to agree on a time limit within which life support will be withdrawn. Help the family to begin their grief work within this period of time. Allow time with the patient to say good-bye.

6. If the family refuses to allow   life-support to be discontinued, notify your supervisor and consult the bioethics committee.

Bibliography

Gellman B. Life Support [Brain Death] Case Rushed into D.C. Court. The Washington Post. 1990 March 10.

Guidelines for the Determination of Death: Report of the Medical Consultants on the Diagnosis of Death to the President's Commission for the Study of Ethical Problems in Medicine and Biomedical and Behavioral Research. Journal of the American Medical Association. 1981 November 13; 246(19): 2184-2186.

Kaufman HH. and Lynn J. Brain Death. Neurosurgery. 1986 November; 19(5):850-856.

Parents want Infant Declared 'Brain Dead' Kept on Respirator, Medical Ethics Advisor. 1990 January; 6(1): 14-16.

Stephenson C. Brain Death in Children: Is there a Difference? Focus on Critical Care. 1987 February; 14(1): 49-56.

Instructional Improvement Tool for Unit

Student feedback/evaluation indicated that I need to improve my classroom presentation by:

Adding Content

1. _____

_____

2. _____

_____

3. _____

_____

Deleting Content

1. _____

_____

2. _____

_____

3. _____

_____

Emphasizing/De-emphasizing the Following Content

1. _____

_____

2. _____

_____

3. _____

_____

Questions students asked that I need to research for the future are:

1. _____

_____

_____

2. _____

_____

3. _____

_____

61
Assessment of Musculoskeletal Function

I. Learning Objectives:

In addition to the learning objectives on page 1831, I want my students to be able to:

1. _____

2. _____

3. _____

II. Top Terms:

1. Atrophy
2. Bursa
3. Crepitus
4. Diaphysis
5. Effusion
6. Hypertrophy
7. Isometric
8. Isotonic
9. Ligaments
10. Osteoporosis
11. Periosteum
12. Sarcomere
13. Synovium
14. Tendons
15. Tonus

III. Collaborative Learning Activities:

Team Discussion Questions/Seminar Topics

1. Explain the interaction between the five factors that help regulate bone formation and bone resorption: stress, vitamin D, parathyroid hormone, calcitonin, and circulation.

2. Describe how blood cells are produced in the bone marrow.

3. Describe some expected musculoskeletal changes that occur with aging.

IV. Critical Thinking Activities

In-Class Team Exercises

Match the function of specific bone tissue listed in Column II with its associated type of bone listed in Column I. (reference page 1832, Chart 61-1)

Column I

_____ 1. bone marrow

_____ 2. osteon

_____ 3. osteoclasts

_____ 4. endosteum

_____ 5. osteoblasts

_____ 6. periosteum

Column II

a. bone formation occurs by the secretion of bone matrix

b. this membrane covers the marrow cavity of long bones

c. this tissue produces red and white blood cells

d. this membrane covers the bone

e. the microscopic functioning unit of mature bone

f. these cells help bone reabsorption and remodeling

Send-Home Assignments

Complete a physical examination of the musculoskeletal system on three individuals that you know: a child under 14 years of age, an adult, and an elderly person over 70 years of age. Document differences in muscle strength, appearance, use, range of motion, and any abnormalities/deformities. Compare and contrast differences among age groups.

62
Management Modalities for Patients with Musculoskeletal Dysfunction

I. Learning Objectives:

In addition to the learning objectives on page 1845, I want my students to be able to:

1. _____

2. _____

3. _____

II. Top Terms:

1. Arthroplasty
2. Atelectasis
3. Avascular Necrosis
4. Capillary Refill
5. Countertraction
6. Meniscectomy

7. Open Reduction
8. Osteoarthritis
9. Osteomyelitis
10. Orthoses
11. Parestheses
12. Volkmann's Contracture

III. Collaborative Learning Activities:

Team Discussion Questions/Seminar Topics

1. Explain, demonstrate, and give the scientific rationale for the process used for turning a patient in a hip spica cast.

2. Explain, demonstrate, and give the scientific rationale for quadriceps and gluteal-setting exercises.

3. Explain why adequate hydration is essential for an orthopedic patient who is immobilized and on bed rest.

IV. Critical Thinking Activities

In-Class Team Exercises

Complete the following chart for each of the following common types of cylindrical casts. (reference page 1848)

Cast Type	Area Covered	Pressure Point	Nursing Assessments	Patient Education
Short Arm Cast				
Long Leg Cast				
Walking Cast				
Body Cast				
Spica Cast				
Hip Spica Cast				

Send-Home Assignments

Read the following case study. Fill in the blanks or circle the correct answer.

Case Study: Total Hip Replacement

Tom is a 62-year-old athletic coach at a high school. Sports activities, especially baseball, have been the focus of his energies since he was in high school and college. Because of prior hip joint injuries and degenerative joint disease, he is scheduled for a total hip replacement. (reference pages 1869-1876)

1. Preoperatively, the nurse assesses the status of the cardiovascular system based on the knowledge that mortality for patients over 60 years is directly related to the complications of: (a) _____ and (b) _____.

2. As part of preoperative teaching the nurse makes the patient aware of four major potential complications of hip replacement:

   a. _____

   b. _____

   c. _____

   d. _____

3. Based on the knowledge that limited hip flexion decreases hip prosthesis dislocation, the nurse knows to:

   a. keep the patient flat in bed with the leg extended.

   b. gatch the knees to decrease the effect of pulling force on the hip.

   c. raise the head of the bed between 30 and 45 degrees.

   d. maintain the patient in semi-Fowler's position.

4. The nurse teaches Tom how to minimize hip extension during transfers and while sitting. She should encourage him to:

   a. rotate the hip inward slightly during sitting to prevent pressure on the external border of the hip.

   b. hyperextend the leg during transfers so the hip socket won't "pop-out."

   c. maintain adduction and flexion when moving around to minimize strain at the surgical site.

   d. always pivot on the unoperated leg to protect the operated leg from unnecessary work.

5. A dislocated prosthesis is evidenced by any of the following five indicators:

   a. _____

   b. _____

   c. _____

   d. _____

   e. _____

6. In assessing postoperative wound drainage, the nurse knows that Tom's drainage of _____ ml in the first 24 hours is within normal range.

    a. 150

    b. 350

    c. 600

    d. 1000

7. The nurse is careful to assess for evidence of deep vein thrombosis which occurs in approximately _____ percent of patients, with a mortality rate up to 3%.

    a. 20

    b. 35

    c. 55

    d. 85

8. Explain the complication, avascular necrosis.

    _____

    _____

CASE STUDY IN PROFESSIONAL COMPETENCY

A 35 year old female patient is admitted to an orthopedic unit where you work as a staff RN. The patient is admitted from the Recovery Room after a reduction of a fibula fracture secondary to a motor vehicle crash. The patient has a cast from her thigh to her toes. The patient progresses normally on the day of surgery, but on her first post-operative day she begins to complain of pain in her casted heel. You note that there is no drainage from the cast and that her toes have good circulation and neurological status. You provide her with the pain medication ordered for her, but this is not adequate to cover her pain. On her second post-operative day, after consultation with the physician, he discontinues the patient's oral pain medication and prescribes a patient-controlled analgesia pump for better pain management. By the third post operative day, the patient is at the upper limit of the pain medication through the PCA pump and still complaining of severe pain in her heel. On that day, you notice a change in her condition. Her temperature has spiked to 101_ F, there is a small amount of drainage at the heel area of her cast) and her toes on the casted foot are edematous and cool.

You page the physician and report your observations. The physician becomes angry and refuses to come to the unit to examine the patient's foot. He accuses you of not knowing how to take care of orthopedic patients and then states that the only reason that the patient has pain is because she has an addictive personality and has become addicted to the pain medication. As evidence he cites the fact, which is true, that the patient's blood alcohol level in the emergency room on admission was 0.12%. Before the physician hangs up on you he tells you that he does not want to hear anything more about this patient's ankle pain.

Discussion:	This is not, strictly speaking, an ethical dilemma. The nursing obligation to protect her patient is clear and there is no countervailing ethical obligation to protect the physician. But the pressure on this nurse not to follow through on her observations about her patient is quite real. The nurse may indeed be placing herself in an angry, confrontational battle with this physician which could lead to some difficult working relationships with him in the future. Nevertheless, the nurse is ethically obligated to intervene in this situation to protect the patient. Indeed, if she does not pursue this matter, she may find herself guilty of neglect and malpractice.
Dilemma:	The obligation to protect the patient is impeded by political and social pressures not to pursue the issue.
Option #1:	Confront the patient with your evidence , denounce the physician as incompetent and urge the patient to another physician.
Rationale:	The patient has a right to know that she is receiving unsafe medical care.
Implications of choosing this option:	The nurse may find herself at cross-purposes with nursing administration, as this action is undoubtedly not consistent with any hospital policy. If wrong about the physician, you will have destroyed the physician-patient relationship, poorly represented the nurses on your unit, and may find yourself sued for slander. The second physician may agree with the first physician. The patient's primary physician will be angry and you may find yourself sued for slander.
Option #2:	Document your information clearly and do not pursue the issue further. The record will speak for itself.
Rationale:	The documentation will help to make the case against the physician while you protect yourself.
Implications of choosing this option:	The patient will not receive the medical attention she needs; she will undoubtedly need to suffer harm before medical chart will be reviewed. The physician may blame you for not notifying him earlier and more forcefully of the patient's problem. Nursing administration may blame you for not pursuing the issue further. You may be liable for malpractice.

Option #3:	Re-verify your information, consult with your peers and your supervisor. Explain to your supervisor why you believe the patient requires medical intervention. Go up the chain of command to the obtain the medical care that the patient needs.
Rationale:	This will produce medical and administrative backing for intervening in the patient's current care and will preserve professional relationships.
Implications of choosing this option:	The patient will receive the medical attention that she needs and professional relationships will be maintained. The physician may be angry at you but administrative support will make it politically difficult for him to express it.

Guidelines for the nurse dealing with an issue of competency:

1. Re-verify your information. Review the chart and note the patient's history, course of illness, present problem, documentation of the present problem, and the present plan of care. Consult with your peers, clinical specialist, and your supervisor to confirm or challenge your conclusions.

2. If your conclusions are verified, document them and attempt again to speak to the physician about your concerns. Document this conversation, including details about information given to the physician.

3. If the physician refuses to intervene in the way you think is necessary for the good of your patient, consult with your supervisor. Describe the information that supports your argument.

4. If the supervisor agrees with your conclusions, she should attempt to speak with the physician. If that fails to bring about the desired intervention, the supervisor can make contacts within the medical chain of command (medical director of the unit, chief of surgery, hospital administrator in charge of medical staff and so on) who can then contact the patient's physician and initiate the required treatment for the patient.

5. Other resources for the nurse in this situation are the Risk Manager and the bioethics committee.

Bibliography

American Nurses' Association. Code for Nurses with Interpretive Statements. Kansas City, Mo., American Nurses' Association, 1985.

American Nurses' Association. Ethics of Safeguarding Client Health and Safety. Ethics in Nursing: Position Statements and Guidelines. Kansas City, Mo., American Nurses' Association, 1988:8-9.

Bandman E. Whistle-Blowers Take Risks to Halt Wrongdoing in Ethical Dilemmas Confronting Nurses. Kansas City, Mo., American Nurses' Association, 1985:18-22.

Edwards BS. When the Physician Won't Give Up. Amer J Nurs. 1993 September; 93(9): 34-37.

Winslow GR. From Loyalty to Advocacy: A new Metaphor for Nursing. Hastings Center Report. 1984 June; 14(3): 32-40.

63

Managing Patients with Musculoskeletal Disorders

I. Learning Objectives:

In addition to the learning objectives on page 1879, I want my students to be able to:

1. _____

2. _____

3. _____

II. Top Terms:

1. Bunion
2. Dupuytren's Contracture
3. Epicondylitis
4. Ganglion
5. Intervertebral Discs

6. Kyphosis
7. Osteogenic
8. Osteoporosis
9. TENS

III. Collaborative Learning Activities:

Team Discussion Questions/Seminar Topics

1. Compare and contrast the clinical manifestations, medical management, and nursing interventions for bursitis and tenosynovitis.

2. Explain the pathophysiology of and latest management techniques for tennis elbow.

3. Explain in detail the relationship between menopause and osteoporosis.

IV. Critical Thinking Activities:

In-Class Team Exercises

1. Develop a patient teaching outline for a 36-year-old mother of six (children range in age from 1 year to 8 years) who suffers from chronic low back pain. Make your instructions specific to her needs. She lives in a split-level house. The kitchen is on the middle level, the washer and dryer are on the lower level, and the children's toy room is in a converted attic area. Try to emphasize modifications for standing, sitting, lying, and lifting. (reference pages 1880-1884)

2. Construct a diet that would provide 1.5 to 2.0 gm of calcium daily for a 60-year-old woman who is moderately active and does not drink milk. The diet should be a weight-reducing diet, since this person is 5 feet 5 inches tall and is 12 pounds overweight. (reference page 1892)

Send-Home Assignments

Review the pictures of common foot deformities found in Figure 63-5, page 1889. Answer the questions below.

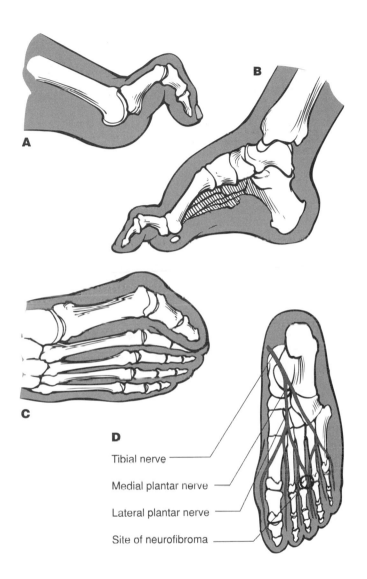

1. Identify each foot ailment and list the associated clinical manifestations.

2. For each ailment, list associated nursing diagnoses.

3. From each diagnosis, draft a nursing plan of care.

4. Broadly explain the medical/surgical management for each ailment.

64

Management of Patients with Musculoskeletal Trauma

I. Learning Objectives:

In addition to the learning objectives on page 1907, I want my students to be able to:

1. _____

2. _____

3. _____

II. Top Terms:

1. Arthroscopic
2. Colles' fracture
3. Ecchymosis
4. Fat Embolis
5. Hemarthrosis

6. Ischemia
7. Pseudoarthrosis
8. Subluxation
9. Tendinitis

III. Collaborative Learning Activities:

Team Discussion Questions/Seminar Topics

1. Describe the concept behind the acronym ICE as it refers to the management of soft tissue injuries.

2. List clinical manifestations commonly associated with fractures and identify a nursing care activity for each clinical manifestation.

3. Compare and contrast the clinical symptoms found with circulatory and neurologic disturbances.

4. Describe recommended sequence of activities necessary for residual limb conditioning.

IV. Critical Thinking Activities:

In-Class Team Exercises

1. Imagine that a classmate has experienced a fracture of the clavicle. Apply a figure-of-8 bandage, and have one of your instructors check it for accurate placement. (reference page 1919 and Figure 64-5)

2. Demonstrate for a classmate the range-of-motion exercises recommended for a patient who has sustained a clavicular fracture. (reference page 1919 and Figure 64-5)

3. Compare and contrast those factors that enhance fracture healing versus those than inhibit healing. (reference pages 1912-1914 and Chart 64-2)

Send-Home Assignments

Complete a nursing care plan for an elderly person who has sustained a hip fracture. Divide your care plan into a preoperative section and a postoperative section. Use the format below. Share your finished paper with your instructor for comment. (reference pages 1925-1928)

Nursing Diagnosis:

Immediate Goal(s):

Intermediate Goal(s):

Long-Term Goal(s):

Nursing Interventions   Expected Outcomes

Instructional Improvement Tool for Unit

Student feedback/evaluation indicated that I need to improve my classroom presentation by:

Adding Content

1. _____
_____

2. _____
_____

3. _____
_____

Deleting Content

1. _____
_____

2. _____
_____

3. _____
_____

Emphasizing/De-emphasizing the Following Content

1. _____
_____

2. _____
_____

3. _____
_____

Questions students asked that I need to research for the future are:

1. _____
_____

2. _____
_____

3. _____
_____

65

Management of Patients with Infectious Diseases

I. Learning Objectives:

In addition to the learning objectives on page 1953, I want my students to be able to:

1. _____

2. _____

3. _____

II. Top Terms:

1. Bacteremia
2. Chlamydia
3. Contagious
4. Epidemiology
5. Epstein-Barr Virus
6. Gonorrhea
7. Herpes Virus
8. MRSA
9. Normal Flora
10. Nosocomial Infection
11. OSHA
12. Portal of Entry
13. Reservoir
14. Septicemia
15. Syphilis

III. Collaborative Learning Activities:

Team Discussion Questions/Seminar Topics

1. Discuss the purpose, location, and role of the Centers for Disease Control.

2. Explain how necrotic tissue is transformed into a cheesy mass in tuberculosis.

3. Describe the nurse's role in preventing and/or managing infectious mononucleosis.

IV. Critical Thinking Activities:

In-Class Team Exercises

Complete the following chart for each of the specific diseases or conditions. (reference pages 1955-1956 and Table 65-1)

Disease or Condition	Organism	Usual Mode of Transmission	Nursing Measures for Prevention of Spread
AIDS			
Gonorrhea			
Chancroid			
Chickenpox			
Cholera			
Hepatitis (food borne)			
Cytomegalovirus Infection			
Hepatitis (blood borne)			
Herpes Simplex			
Impetigo			
Legionnaire's Disease			
Measles			
Meningitis			
Pneumocystis Pneumonia			
Rabies			
Rubella (blood borne)			
Syphilis			
Tetanus			
Tuberculosis			

Send-Home Assignments

Examine Figure 65-1 below. For each of the six links in the infection cycle, describe specific nursing interventions that can be used to break transmission. (reference pages 1954-1957)

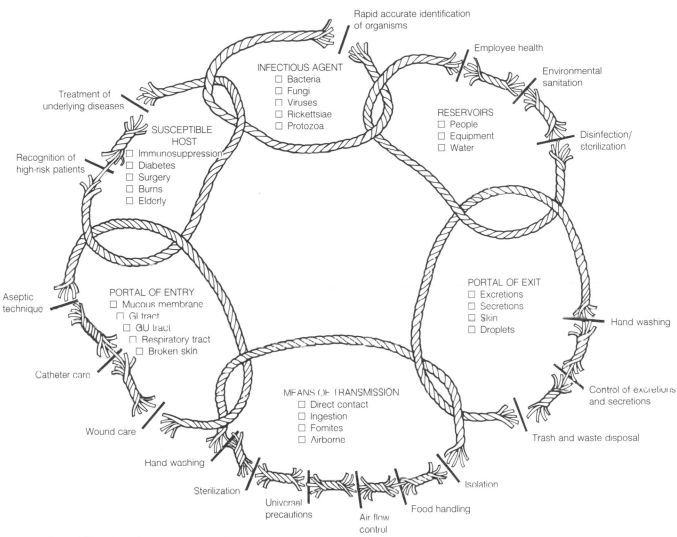

Specific Nursing Interventions

Link #1: Infectious Agent

1. Patient education about immunization (Example) _____

2. _____

3. _____

Link #2: Reservoirs

1. _____

2. _____

3. _____

Link #3: Portal of Exit

1. _____

2. _____

3. _____

Link #4: Means of Transmission

1. _____

2. _____

3. _____

Link #5: Portal of Entry

1. _____

2. _____

3. _____

Link #6: Susceptible Host

1. _____

2. _____

3. _____

66
Emergency Nursing

I. Learning Objectives:

In addition to the learning objectives on page 1999, I want my students to be able to:

1. _____

2. _____

3. _____

II. Top Terms:

1. Anaphylactic Reaction
2. Antitoxin
3. Carboxyhemoglobin
4. Endotracheal Intubation
5. Erythema

6. Hypercarbia
7. Hypothermia
8. Hypoxia
9. Lavage

III. Collaborative Learning Activities:

Team Discussion Questions/Seminar Topics

1. Describe three symptoms that a nurse would expect to see in someone who is experiencing post-traumatic stress disorder.

2. Explain what a nurse should do for both acid and corrosive poisoning both at the scene of the action and at the emergency room.

3. List the priorities of nursing interventions with supporting rationales for the treatment of frostbite.

IV. Critical Thinking Activities:

In-Class Team Exercises

1. Work in teams of two. Each person needs to palpate the seven pressure points used to control hemorrhage on their partner. (reference pages 2010-2012 and Figure 66-3)

2. Have a volunteer bring in the MAST trouser. Take turns having each person demonstrate how to apply it and explain the rationale for its use (reference pages 2016-2018 and Figure 66-4)

3. For each of the drugs listed below, identify the recommended nursing interventions with supporting rationales. (reference pages 2027-2031 and Table 66-1)

Drug	Clinical Manifestations	Nursing Interventions
Cocaine		
Opium		
Morphine		
Secanal		
Amphetamine		
"LSD"		
Valium		

Send-Home Assignments

Develop a nursing care plan for a 16-year-old high school student who was brought into the emergency department by her parents. She had been raped on her way home from cheerleading practice. On admission she was withdrawn and would only talk about the situation with her mother. (reference pages 2036-2037)

Nursing Diagnosis:

Immediate Goal(s):

Intermediate Goal(s):

Long-Term Goal(s):

Nursing Interventions   Expected   Outcomes

ETHICAL QUESTION: SHOULD A JEHOVAH'S WITNESS PATIENT RECEIVE LIFE-SAVING BLOOD TRANSFUSIONS AGAINST HIS WISHES?

Discussion: The purpose of emergency departments is to provide life-saving treatment for patients. Jehovah's Witnesses are a sect of Christians who agree to aggressive medical treatment in case of illness or trauma, but who consistently refuse any blood or blood products because of their unique interpretation of the Bible. Should a viable and potentially salvageable Jehovah's Witness patient suffering from an acute blood loss be allowed to die because of a request based on religious beliefs if a relatively easy and accessible treatment (that is, blood transfusions) could save his life?

Dilemma: The patient's right to refuse treatment conflicts with the professional obligation to help the patient (autonomy versus beneficence).

Arguments that Jehovah's Witnesses SHOULD receive lifesaving transfusions against their will: The professional obligation to help the patient is more important than the patent's right to refuse treatment. Religious beliefs are not as important as saving lives.

Implications of choosing this position: The lives of some patients who otherwise would have died without blood transfusions will be saved. Jehovah's Witnesses whose lives are saved by blood transfusions may find themselves ostracized from their church and family and may believe that they cannot go to heaven. Giving blood transfusions against the patient's will shows disrespect for minority religious beliefs. The patient may suffer side effects from the blood transfusions including hepatitis or HIV infection. The patient may die despite the blood transfusion. The professionals who transfuse the patient over his objections may find themselves liable for malpractice or assault.

Arguments that Jehovah's Witnesses SHOULD NOT receive blood transfusions if they refuse them: The patient's right to refuse treatment is more important than the professional's desire to save the patient's life. Patients do not lose their right to make health care choices just because those choices are based on religious beliefs.

Implications of choosing this position: Patients will die who would have survived with blood transfusions. Professionals may feel guilty about patients' deaths from lack of blood transfusions. Religious beliefs are respected. Some patients will survive despite the lack of blood transfusions.

Possible compromise position: Uphold the right of patients to refuse life-saving treatment based on religious beliefs except when minor children and pregnant women are involved, under the theory that unborn babies and children have not "chosen" the Jehovah's Witness religion. This has been the opinion of most trial courts in the United States. This exception for pregnant women, of course, raises ethical questions about the rights of pregnant women versus non- pregnant women.

Guidelines for the nurse caring for a Jehovah's Witness patient with a life-threatening need for a blood transfusion:

1. Explore the issue of blood transfusion with the patient. Explain the risks and benefits of the treatment. The patient should be able to give an informed consent for blood or no blood. Document your discussion and the patient's decision clearly in the patient's chart.

2. If the patient refuses a blood transfusion, notify the physician. Encourage the physician to talk to the patient and explain again the risks and benefits of treatment with and without blood transfusions. Again, document this discussion and the patient's decision in the patient's chart.

3. Not every Jehovah's Witness will refuse blood transfusions. If the patient agrees to a blood transfusion, document this clearly in the chart and proceed with the transfusion as ordered. Keep in mind that the patient may not want to share this information with his family or friends. Talk with the patient about this. You may need to curb visitors to the patient during the transfusion. Talk with the patient and physician about how to handle requests from family members about the specifics of the patient's treatment and agree upon a plan.

4. If the patient refuses a blood transfusion, document this clearly in the patient's chart. Notify your supervisor. Consider alternative forms of treatment acceptable to the patient, for example, infusion of volume expanders or vasopressors, or both. Discuss treatment of the underlying bleeding source with the physician.

5. If the physician orders a blood transfusion despite the patient's refusal, notify your supervisor, consult with the institution's Risk Management office, and initiate an immediate Bioethics Committee consultation.

Bibliography

Devine RJ. Save the Body, Lose the Soul: Catholic Healthcare Professionals Should Respect Jehovah's Witnesses' Right to Refuse a Transfusion. Health Progress. 1989 June:68-72.

Dixon JL. and Smalley MG. Jehovah's Witnesses: The Surgical/Ethical Challenge. Journal of the American Medical Association. 1981 November 27; 286(21): 2471-2472.

Jehovah's Witnesses and the Question of Blood New York. Watchtower Bible and Tract Society of New York, Inc., 1977.

Jonsen AR. Commentary (on Vinickey, et. al.): Jehovah's Witnesses and Blood. The Journal of Clinical Ethics. 1990 Spring; 1(1) :71-72.

Macklin R. The Inner Workings of an Ethics Committee: Latest Battle over Jehovah's Witnesses. The Hastings Center Report. 1988 February-March; 18(1):15-20.

Reed NA. Commentary (on Vinickey, et. al.): Response from Jehovah's Witnesses. The Journal of Clinical Ethics. 1990 Spring; 1(1):72-74.

Vinicky, JK. et. al. The Jehovah's Witness and Blood: New Perspectives on an Old Dilemma. The Journal of Clinical Ethics. 1990 Spring; 1(1):65-71.

Instructional Improvement Tool for Unit

Student feedback/evaluation indicated that I need to improve my classroom presentation by:

Adding Content

1. _____

   _____

2. _____

   _____

3. _____

   _____

Deleting Content

1. _____

   _____

2. _____

   _____

3. _____

   _____

Emphasizing/De-emphasizing the Following Content

1. _____

   _____

2. _____

   _____

3. _____

   _____

Questions students asked that I need to research for the future are:

1. _____

   _____

   _____

2. _____

   _____

3. _____

   _____

Answer Key

Based upon the individual responses to most of the exercises, specific answers are only provided for case studies, multiple-choice responses and sample flow charts.

Chapter 1

CQI Cause and Effect Diagram: Delayed Medication
Possible Causes

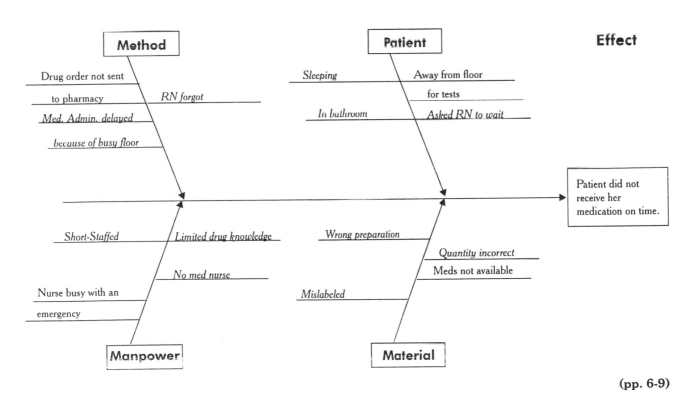

(pp. 6-9)

Chapter 8

Flow Chart:Representative Pathophysiologic Process:
Hypertensive Heart Disease

Decreased Renal   =   ↑ Renin
Blood Flow

                 ↑ Angiotensin I   } =   ↑ Blood Pressure

                 ↑ Angiotensin II   ↑ Aldosterone   } =   ↑ Increased
                                                   ↑ Retention of Sodium   Extracellular
                                                         and Water   Fluid

Increased   =   ↑ Blood flow
Extracellular Fluid

                 ↑ to the Heart   } =   ↑ Cardiac
                                       ↑ Output   } =   ↑ Increased Stroke
                                                                     Volume

Increased Stroke   =   ↑ Peripheral
Volume

                 ↑ Resistance   } =   ↑ Left Ventricular

                                       ↑ Emptying   } =   ↑ Increased
                                       ↑   Pulmonary
                                                                      Activity

Increased   =   ↑ Pulmonary
Pulmonary Activity   Edema

(pp. 103-104)

Chapter 9

Flow Chart: Sympathetic-Adrenal-Medullary Response

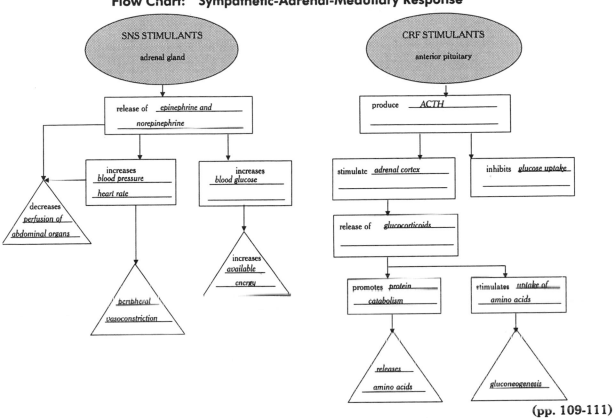

(pp. 109-111)

Chapter 14

Case Study: Arthroscopy

1. a

2. a

3. d

4. d

(pp. 238-244)

Three Column Matching

1.	d	a.	V
2.	e	b.	IV
3.	f	c.	III
4.	a	d.	II
5.	b	e.	VI
6.	c	f.	I

(pp. 206-209)

Chapter 15

Flow Chart: Hypovolemic Shock

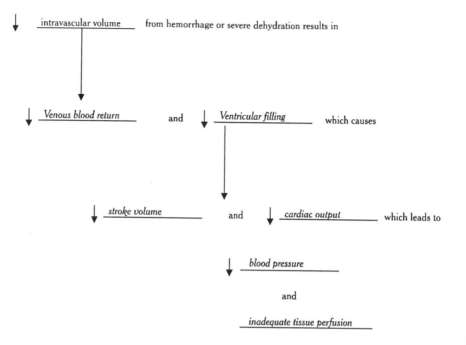

intravascular volume   from hemorrhage or severe dehydration results in

↓ Venous blood return   and   ↓ Ventricular filling   which causes

↓ stroke volume   and   ↓ cardiac output   which leads to

↓ blood pressure

and

inadequate tissue perfusion

(pp. 255-257)

Case Study: Septic Shock

1. Escherichia Coli

2. 40% and 90%

3. a. urine

    b. blood

    c. sputum

    d. wound drainage

4. a. aggressive fluid replacement

    b. antibiotic pharmacotherapy

    c. crystalloids

    d. colloids

5. Cardiovascular overload and pulmonary edema

6. 4-12 cm H_2O

(pp. 262-263)

Chapter 16

Case Study: Cancer of the Lung

1. d

2. a. disease progression

    b. immune competence

    c. increased incidence of infection

    d. delayed tissue repair

    e. diminished functional ability

3. a. fear

    b. apprehension

    c. fatigue

    d. anger

    e. social isolation

4. c

5. a. answer questions and concerns

    b. identify resources and support persons

    c. communicate and share concerns

    d. help frame questions for the physician

6. infection

7. Pseudomonas aeruginosa and Escherichia coli

8. b   **(pp. 290-297)**

Chapter 18

Case Study: Pressure Ulcers

1. d

2. b

3. d

4. d

(pp. 329-335)

Case Study: Assisted Ambulation: Crutches

1. b

2. b

3. c

4. b

(pp. 334-340)

Chapter 20

Case Study: Spinal Anesthesia

1. d

2. d

3. d

(pp. 382-384 [Table 20-6])

Case Study: Malignant Hyperthermia

1. b

2. a

3. d

(pp. 388-389)

Chapter 21

Case Study: Hypovolemic Shock

1. b

2. b

3. a

4. a

5. b

(pp. 403-405)

Chapter 23

Case Study: The Common Cold

1. a. nasal congestion

   b. sore throat

   c. sneezing

   d. malaise

    e.   fever

    f.   chills

    g.   headache

    h.   muscle aches

2. a

3. d

4. d

5. d

6. a.   rest

    b.   adequate fluids

    c.   nasal decongestants

    d.   Vitamin C

    e.   expectorants

7. Tells Carol that antibiotics do not affect the virus.   **(p. 462)**

Chapter 24

Case Study: Tuberculosis

1. b

2. b

3. d

4. b

5. c

6. c   **(pp. 495-501 [Figures 24-2 and 24-3 and Table 24-2])**

Chapter 26

Case Study: Cardiac Assessment for Chest Pain

1. d

2. c

3. d   **(pp. 598-599)**

Chapter 27

Case Study: Permanent Pacemaker

1. Yes. Heart rate can vary as much as five beats above or below the preset rate.

2. a. bleeding, b. hematoma formation, and c. infection

3. infection; maintaining a clean incision site

4. a. pacemaker model

   b. date and time of insertion

   c. stimulation threshold

   d. pacer rate

   e. incision appearance

   f. patient tolerance

5.

Goals	Nursing Activities	Expected Outcomes
a. Absence of infection	a. Sterile wound care	a. Free of infection
b. Adherence to a self-care program	b. Patient teaching	b. Adheres to a self-care program
c. Maintenance of pacemaker function	c. Patient teaching	c. Maintains pacemaker function

6. a. Normal temperature, WBCs within normal range and no evidence of redness or swelling at insertion site

   b. Understands sign and symptoms of infection and knows when to seek medical attention

   c. Assesses pulse rate at regular intervals and experiences no abrupt changes in pulse rate or rhythm

(pp. 629-633)

Chapter 28

Case Study: Pulmonary Edema

1. cardiac disease

2. a

3. d

4. b

5. d

6. d

(pp. 654-661)

Chapter 29

Case Study: Acute Pericarditis

1. a

2. Pain related to inflammation of the pericardium

3. d

4. a. Analgesics, b. Antibiotics, and c. Corticosteroids

5. Left sternal edge in the fourth intercostal space

6. a. Freedom from pain and b. Experiences absence of complications

(pp. 690-692)

Chapter 30

Case Study: Coronary Artery Bypass Graft Surgery

1. d

2. d

3. c

4. c

(pp. 696-698)

Chapter 31   Schematic: Pathophysiology of Essential Hypertension

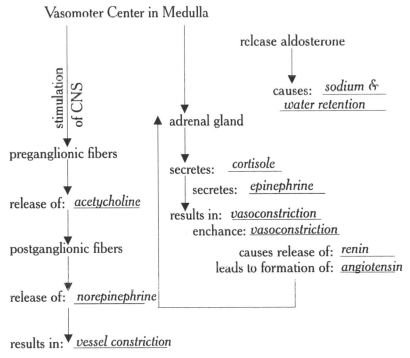

Vasomoter Center in Medulla

release aldosterone

causes: _sodium & water retention_

stimulation of CNS

adrenal gland

preganglionic fibers

secretes: _cortisole_

secretes: _epinephrine_

release of: _acetycholine_

results in: _vasoconstriction_
enchance: _vasoconstriction_

postganglionic fibers

causes release of: _renin_
leads to formation of: _angiotensin_

release of: _norepinephrine_

results in: _vessel constriction_

(pp. 741-751)

Case Study: Thrombophlebitis

1. d

2. a

3. b

4. b

5. d

(pp. 752-757)

Chapter 32

Case Study: Leukemia

1. hematopoietic stem cell

2. immature blast cells

3. d

4. b

5. b

(pp. 791-792)

Chapter 34

Case Study: Cancer of the Mouth

1. The typical lesion in oral cancer is a painless, indurated (hardened) ulcer with raised edges

2. d

3. d

4. a

5. Resectional surgery, radiation therapy and chemotherapy are considered effective.

6. c

7. d

(pp. 837-841)

Chapter 35

Case Study: Total Parenteral Nutrition

1. b

2. c

3. c

4. d

5. d

(pp. 874-879)

Chapter 37

```
      F         M       5         C
      I         E   F   F   L   U   E   N   T
      S         G       U         L             V
S   T   O   M   A                 E             A             C
      U         C                 R             L             R
      L       D   O   R   B   O   R   Y   M   U   S           O
      A         O                               A             H
                L                               L             N'
      C   O   R   N           L   A   X   A   T   I   V   E   S
      E                                         E             A
      A                 E           T   P   N
                        C                   E
P   E   R   I   T   O   N   I   T   I   S
                        L                   M
                        I                   U
                                            S
```

Chapter 38

In-Class Exercise

1. e

2. f

3. a

4. b

5. g

6. c

7. d

(pp. 971-972, Figure 38-5)

Chapter 40

Case Study: Hyperparathyroidism

1. a

2. a

3. a. apathy

   b. fatigue

   c. muscular weakness

   d. nausea

   e. vomiting

   f. constipation

   g. hypertension

   h. cardiac dysrhythmias

4. renal damage subsequent to the precipitation of calcium phosphate resulting in renal stones.

5. d

6. b

7. c

(pp. 1091-1092)

Chapter 43

Case Study: Ileal Conduit

1. d

2. b

3. a

4. d

5. d
(pp. 1217-1220 [Figure 43-7])

Chapter 45

Case Study: Pelvic Inflammatory Disease

1. (a) uterus, (b) fallopian tubes, (c) ovaries, (d) pelvic peritoneum, and (e) pelvic vascular system

2. (a) acute, (b) subacute, (c) recurrent, (d) chronic, (e) localized, and (f) widespread

3. a

4. Gonorrhea and Chlamydia

5. (a) ectopic pregnancy, (b) infertility, (c) recurrent pelvic pain, and (d) recurrent disease

6. Localized: (a) vaginal discharge, (b) lower abdominal pain, (c) and tenderness after menses. Generalized: (a) fever, (b) general malaise, (c) anorexia, (d) nausea, (e) headache, and (f) vomiting.

7. Use Chart 45-3 as a guide.
(pages 1278-1280)

Case Study: Herpes Genitalis

1. d

2. a

3. c

4. (a) mouth, (b) oropharynx, (c) mucosal surface, (d) vagina, and (e) cervix

5. drying at room temperature

6. Acyclovir

7. (a) Pain related to the presence of genital lesions, (b) risk for recurrence of infection or spread of infection, and (c) anxiety and distress related to embarrassment.
(pages 1274-1275)

Chapter 47

Case Study: The Patient Undergoing Prostatectomy

1. Assessment of general health status and establishment of optimum renal function.

2. Acute urinary retention develops and damages the urinary tract and collecting system.

3. d

4. Stricture formation and retrograde ejaculation

5. Hemorrhage, clot formation, catheter obstruction, and sexual dysfunction

6. Damage to the pudendal nerves may cause impotence

7. Anxiety related to the inability to void, pain related to bladder distention, and knowledge deficit about factors related to the problem and the treatment protocol

8. Warm compresses to the pubis and sitz baths can help relieve spasms

9. Prolonged sitting increases intra-abdominal pressure and increases the possibility of bleeding

10. Teach the patient to tense the perineal muscles by pressing the buttocks together, holding the position for 15-20 seconds, and then relaxing. **(pages 1341-1347)**

Chapter 49

Identifying Patterns

1. B-cell deficiencies (p. 1382)

2. CVID (pp. 1382-1384)

3. antimicrobial therapy (pp. 1382-1384)

4. hypocalcemia and tetany (p. 1384)

5. excess occurrences of lysis (p. 1385)

Chapter 52

In-Class Exercises: Laboratory Significance

1. a
2. d
3. e

4. a

5. f

6. b
                                                            (pp. 1450-1451 [Table 52-1])

In-Class Exercises: Rheumatic Diseases

1. c

2. d

3. a

4. e

5. b

6. g

7. c

8. f

9. e

10. d   **(p. 1444 [Chart 52-1])**

Chapter 53

Matching

Part I   Part II

    1. b   1. d

    2. a   2. c

    3. c   3. a

    4. d   4. e

    5. e   5. b   **(pp. 1486-1488 [Chart 53-2])**

Chapter 54

Case Study: Acne Vulgaris

1. open and closed comedones, papules, pustules, modules and cysts

2. d

3. c

4. Benzoyl Peroxide has an antibacterial effect because it suppresses Propionibacterium acnes, depresses sebum production and helps breakdown comedone plugs.

5. Vitamin A clears up the keratin plugs from the pilosebaceous ducts by speeding up cellular turnover and forcing the comedone out of the skin.

6. c

7. a

8. scarring and infection

(pp. 1505-1509)

Chapter 55

Flow Chart: Systemic Response to Burn Injury

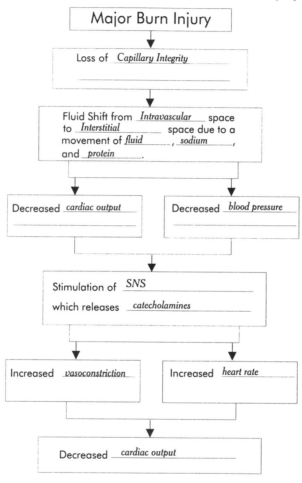

(pp. 1546-1549)

Chapter 56

Case Study: Cataract Surgery

1. smoking, diabetes mellitus, alcohol abuse, and inadequate intake of antioxidant vitamins over time

2. diminished visual acuity, glare, and functional impairment due to loss of vision

3. a grayish pearly haze in the pupil

4. d

5. extracapsular extraction

6. c

7. c   (pp. 1612-1615)

Chapter 57

In-Class Exercise: Unscramble the Word

1. | C | O | C | H | L | E | A |

2. | A | U | R | I | C | L | E |

3. | C | E | R | U | M | E | N |

4. | M | A | L | L | E | U | S |

5. | I | N | C | U | S |

6. | E | I | G | H | T | H |

7. | L | A | B | R | Y | I | N | T | H |

8. | T | Y | M | P | A | N | I | C |

(pp. 1644-1646 [Chart 57-1])

Chapter 61

Matching Test

1. c   4. b

2. e   5. a

3. f   6. d   (p. 1832, Chart 61-1)

Chapter 62

Case Study: Total Hip Replacement

1. deep vein thrombosis and pulmonary embolism

2. dislocation of the hip prosthesis, excessive wound drainage, thromboembolism, and infection

3. c

4. d

5. leg shortening, inability to move the leg, malalignment, abnormal rotation and increased localized discomfort

6. b

7. c

8. Avascular necrosis is bone death caused by loss of blood supply   **(pp. 1896-1876)**